I0758318

The New Cleanse: A Fresh Restorative Program for Full Body Detoxification

The New Cleanse: A Fresh Restorative Program for Full Body Detoxification

Copyright © 2023 by **Omolola Habib (NMD)**
All rights reserved. No part of this publication may be reproduced, distributed, or transmitted in any form or by any means, including photocopying, recording, or other electronic or mechanical methods, without the prior written permission of the publisher, except in the case of brief quotations embodied in critical reviews and certain other noncommercial uses permitted by copyright law

Table of Content

Introduction

In today's modern world, we live in an environment flooded with toxins. From pollutants in the air we breathe to pesticides on our foods to chemicals in our cleaning and beauty products, our bodies are constantly bombarded. Many of these substances make their way into our tissues and bloodstream, creating what is termed our "toxic load" - essentially all of the foreign and harmful compounds accumulating inside us.

This gradual builds up of toxins can begin to cause dysfunction in the body and mind. Often the signs are subtle at first - low energy levels, weight gain, skin irritation, headaches, and so on. Over years or decades, higher toxic exposure has been linked to more concerning outcomes like hormone disorders, autoimmune diseases, infertility issues, neurological conditions, and some cancers. Our rising toxic burden simply should not be ignored.

While Western medicine frequently attempts to override symptoms with drugs or surgery, the root cause often lies in imbalance and intoxication at a cellular level. *A true restoration of health and vibrancy means getting to the source by removing what is weighing us down - toxic accumulation - and naturally rebalancing internal systems.*

Why Detoxification Matters

Detoxification refers to the body's innate mechanisms for neutralizing and clearing out foreign substances and waste products. Organs like the liver, kidneys, digestive tract, lungs, and skin work around the clock to transform toxins into less harmful forms that can then be eliminated. Our vitality and lifespan quite literally depend on these critical detoxification pathways operating smoothly.

However, faced with a mounting onslaught of toxins from our unhealthy modern lifestyles, our natural detox systems eventually become overburdened and congested. Toxins start accumulating faster than they can be cleared out, leading to inflammatory and free radical damage. Consequently, our risk of chronic illness rises significantly over time.

Engaging in periodic cleansing programs gives our detox organs a chance "reset", restore proper functioning, and catch up on the toxin backlog by entering a therapeutic state of enhanced elimination. Essentially, we hit control-alt-delete for the body!

Limitations of Popular Cleanses

Various cleanses and "detox diets" have surged in popularity over recent years as more people grow concerned about toxicity. However, many of the mainstream programs are limited in scope or even counterproductive.

For instance:

- **Juice cleanses** supply vital nutrients but deprive complex carbohydrates needed for balanced energy and gut health.

- **Master cleanses** based only on lemon juice, maple syrup, cayenne pepper and water provide no meaningful nutrition and are not sustainable.

- **Enemas and colonics** flush the gastrointestinal tract but fail to address systemic toxicity.

- **Fasting/starvation cleanses** overstress the organs and metabolism leading to loss of muscle.

The most effective cleanse is one that holistically supports ALL the channels of detoxification in the body.

Introducing The New Cleanse

The New Cleanse program outlined in this book goes beyond traditional concepts or notions of detoxing and cleansing. I have designed a comprehensive 21 day protocol utilizing evidence-based strategies to maximize toxin removal while maintaining optimal nutrition status.

The multi-phase system includes:

- Preparation period to reduce exposure and prime detox organs

- Supported fasts and structured refeeding for cell regeneration

- Time-restricted eating patterns to promote elimination

- Targeted supplement regimens to upregulate natural detox enzymes

- Specific foods, juices and lifestyle tips to drive key detox pathways

- Guidance to rebalance gut flora and support immunity

- Recipes and meals focused on the highest quality nutrient-dense whole foods

The program can be customized and adapted to suit individual needs, with troubleshooting guidance provided. Experts interviews are featured throughout the book to provide diverse insights into various detox mechanisms and cutting edge science.

Who Can Benefit?

This cleanse regimen can benefit anyone looking to hit the health reset button after prolonged periods of toxic exposure and mismanaged lifestyle habits. Whether you aim to promote weight loss, improve complexion, reduce inflammation, balance hormones, or prevent chronic disease, removing the body's toxic burden is the first step.

Particularly however, The New Cleanse can be especially restorative for those suffering with:

- Autoimmune conditions

- Frequent infections

- Skin disorders

- Fatigue or low energy

- Obesity

- Diabetes

- Headaches/migraines

- Mental fog

- And more...

If you find your current health limiting your quality of life, struggle with mysterious symptoms, have plateaued with other treatments, or used predecessors of this cleanse before - *embarking on The New Cleanse may provide you with profound benefits.*

While results can never be guaranteed, I invite you to join me over the next 21 days as we explore and experience the transformative power of holistic detoxification. By removing accumulated toxins and restarting our body's purification systems, we can begin to walk the path back to optimal wellness.

Part I: Understanding Detoxification

Before we launch into the specifics of our 21-day cleansing program, it is vital we build a foundational understanding of what detoxification means and how it works in the body. Cleansing goes far beyond just following protocols blindly or choking down funny tasting drinks! Lasting transformation relies on aligning with the body's innate intelligence.

We must remember that our cells, tissues and organs have a spectacular inborn capacity to self-regulate and heal when provided with the right inputs. However, the key stimuli to activate many of these self-repair processes involves first clearing out the impurities and toxins congesting the terrain. *Essentially by removing interference and toxicity we allow health to naturally flourish.*

In Part I of this book, we will cover:

- Defining detoxification pathways and mechanisms

- Cataloguing common toxins and assessing your personal toxic load

- Investigating the wide-ranging impact of toxicity from subtle to severe

- Mapping the key organs (liver, gut, kidneys, skin) involved in cleansing processes along with their ideal functioning state

- Understanding elimination channels like bowel movements, urination, respiration, and sweating

- Appreciating the massive filtering capacities our bodies inherently possess when not obstructed

Arming yourself with knowledge in these areas will allow you to dive into the cleanse from an empowered perspective. *The practices will transform from a mysterious ritual into an intuitive collaboration with your body's wisdom.* My goal is that through education and experience you will finish the 21 days with an expanded awareness of how to support lifelong detoxification for sustainable wellbeing.

We kick off Part I by defining why toxic accumulation matters in the modern world and how it can insidiously undermine health over time if left unaddressed.

Chapter 1: Why We Need to Detox

We live in an unprecedented age of toxic exposure that our ancestors could have never imagined. On top of natural toxins found in our environment like molds or heavy metals, humans have introduced over 100,000 novel synthetic chemicals into the world since the industrial era began. Our modern lifestyles bombard us with hazardous substances on a daily basis. This creates a dilemma our bodies were not designed to handle at such immense levels of contamination.

Toxins essentially represent foreign substances that the body struggles to process and eliminate effectively. The accumulation of unmanaged toxins then sparks a cascade of consequences. Even at low doses, these chemicals and waste products interfere with normal physiology. Organs, glands, tissues, cells, proteins, DNA and more become disrupted. Given the fundamental role homeostasis plays in life, uncontrolled toxicity eventually leads to the breakdown of health.

Simply look at the exponential rise of numerous chronic and degenerative illnesses correlating to the explosion of industrial pollutants. The staggering statistics linked to disorders like obesity, diabetes, infertility, Alzheimer's, ADHD, autoimmunity, and cancer make a compelling case that we face a modern toxicity epidemic. *Our collective toxic burden is catching up to us quickly.*

We each have a decision to either continue accumulating toxins until they manifest into diagnosable diseases, or to regularly clear out hazardous exposures before they cause progressive harm. The New Cleanse solution outlined in this book provides a way to proactively and preventatively take control of your health trajectory.

Categories of Toxins

To appreciate why rigorous detoxification habits matter today, we must first survey the most common toxins that endanger us:

Environmental Pollutants - Pesticides, heavy metals, VOCs, combustion byproducts, plasticizers, and industrial chemicals. Exposure through air, water, soil.

Medications - Residues building up from drugs. Side effects disrupting physiology.

Food Chemicals - Preservatives, colorings, flavorings, pesticides. Burden on detox organs.

Metabolic Waste - Ammonia, free radicals, advanced glycation endproducts. Byproducts of respiration.

Pathogens - Bacterial, viral, fungal. Can release toxic byproducts.

Stress Hormones - Catecholamines and cortisol. Impact gene expression, accelerate aging.

This list while not comprehensive, highlights the diversity of toxic agents that find their way into our environment and subsequently our bodies. Their cumulative impact slowly sabotages wellness from a grassroots level.

And while nature has brilliantly outfitted us with defense mechanisms to neutralize threats, our detoxification systems now face severe overexertion. Our organs simply cannot keep pace with the exponential rise of unnatural toxicity créated in the modern world. Hence the necessity to consciously support your body's cleansing abilities through programs like The New Cleanse.

Toxicity By The Numbers

Some statistics to put the growing toxicity crisis into perspective:

- Over **9 million** deaths annually linked to pollution according to Lancet Commission report

- Developed nations testing reveals **average** of 110 synthetic chemicals in blood and urine that were absent a century ago

- **170%** increase in US autism rates correlating directly to mass introduction of glyphosate and aluminum adjuvant in vaccines

- Up to **5 billion** pounds of toxic chemicals released into environment yearly just in US

These mind-boggling numbers showcase why periodic cleansing is not just a nice extra, but an outright necessity today. Without structured detox, the buildup persists every year.

And the impact of all these chemicals remains largely understudied. But based on the research we do have, an incredibly high price is being paid in the currency of human health.

Hidden Half-Life

One reason toxicity easily escapes our awareness involves the problem of **bioaccumulation** - when the body cannot excrete contaminants as quickly as they enter tissues through exposure. Toxins then progressively stockpile with cumulative damage accruing over months or years before pathology or symptoms arise.

For example, the half-life of glyphosate (Roundup) averages around 22 days. This means every 22 days, 50% has been eliminated while 50% remains stored. Now imagine constant re-exposure through food over months and years. Accumulation gradually enables cellular disruption. Hence the lag time between exposure and diagnosis with chronic conditions.

Without conscious detox habits however, the storage process continues indefinitely resulting in gradual multi-system breakdown. *The poison eventually becomes identifiable only when the disproportionate disease manifests - which represents the tip of a much deeper iceberg.*

Chapter 2: How Toxins Build Up and The Effects on Your Body

Now that we have defined the scope of our contamination woes from the exploding spectrum of toxins in modern times, next we will explore how exactly these hazardous substances make their way inside us and subsequently cause damage after taking up residence.

Understanding the vectors of transmission into the body along with perpetrator toxins and their myriad effects allows us to contextualize why dedicated cleansing periods offer such profound benefits. Essentially we can map how toxins enter, store, disrupt function, and spread inflammation - which sets the stage for why an intensive detox reboot hits the reset button on lagging health and vitality.

Routes of Exposure

Exogenous toxins from our external environment primarily access the body through the following portals:

Gastrointestinal Tract - Digestion of contaminated food/drink or poor microbial flora

Lungs - Inhalation of gases, chemicals, particulate matter

Skin - Absorption of pathogens, allergens plus personal care products

Nose/Eyes - Particulate transmission into bloodstream

Ears - Environmental chemicals traversing external membranes

Urogenital - Unsafe intimate products, yeast overgrowth

Without conscious prevention habits, studies show the average person now harbors over **700 synthetic contaminants** coursing through our tissues and cells from combinatorial exposure! Our filtering organs face severe encumbrance trying to manage this "chemical soup" effectively.

Storage and Bioaccumulation

Once various toxins access our insides, they undergo storage and accumulation through processes like:

Fat Cell Deposits - Lipophilic (fat-loving) chemicals accumulate in adipose tissue like DDT, dioxins, PCBs

Liver and Gallbladder - Fat soluble toxins and hormone metabolites are concentrated here

Arterial Plaque - Heavy metals embed in atheroma debris inside blood vessels

Joints and Bones - Heavy metals replace calcium and lead to degeneration

Brain - Lipophilic toxins + heavy metals accumulate with neurological decline

This highlights why targeted cleansing periods prove so invaluable - we disrupt this gradual bioaccumulation to reduce body burden over time before pathology sets in from cellular impairment.

Cycles of Toxicity

On top of external contamination adding continuously to the total toxic load, we must appreciate the self-perpetuating cycles that amplify the agenda of pre-existing toxins:

Compromised Biotransformation Pathways - Overwhelmed liver, kidneys, unable regulate toxins

Lipid Peroxidation - Free radical cascades degenerate cell membranes

Intestinal Dysbiosis - Imbalanced gut flora release endotoxins into bloodstream

Yeast and Parasite Overgrowth - Microbes encourage inflammation + leaky gut

Hormone Imbalance - Poor excretion leads to excess estrogen, cortisol imbalance

Oxidative Stress - Free radical damage accrues exponentially

Without periodic cleansing, these vicious cycles accelerate the degradation process. The New Cleanse interrupt this downward spiral to restore optimal functioning.

Clinical Effects of Toxicity

The precise damage instigated will vary based on individual toxin exposure, dose, duration, genetics, and lifestyle factors. However categorically, researchers divide the primary chaos induced by bioaccumulation into:

1. Altered Biochemistry - Enzymes dysregulation, inflammation, mitochondrial dysfunction

2. Endocrine Disruption - Hormone imbalance, infertility, reproductive disorders

3. Neurotoxicity - Degeneration of neurons, destruction of myelin

4. Immune Dysfunction - Autoimmunity, allergies, frequent infections

5. DNA Mutations / Cancer - Interference with DNA signaling, uncontrolled replication

Generally, toxicity sparks **oxidative stress** which pulls the rug out from normal metabolic function. Our risk then rises exponentially for numerous common afflictions:

Major Diseases Linked to Toxicity

Autoimmune Disease - Pollutants interact with genetics to trigger self-attack via inflammation and tissue damage.

Obesity + Diabetes - Obesogens reprogram endocrine pathways leading to insulin resistance and weight gain over time

Atherosclerosis - Oxidized LDL, endotoxins, heavy metals drive plaque accumulation in arteries

Infertility - Endocrine disruptors + contaminants interfere with reproductive hormones plus fetal development

Neurodegeneration - Environmental toxins assault neurons and promote plaque formation over decades

Cancer - DNA damage from toxins, nutrient depletion for tumor suppression, carcinogens

Astoundingly age-adjusted cancer rates have exploded over 25% just since the 1990s when GMOs, wireless technology and aggressive chemical expansion all rapidly accelerated!

Beyond specific diseases though, because our cells bathe in this circulating chemical mix disrupting homeostasis, **no organ system avoids consequence.** Diffuse symptoms like fatigue, headaches, rashes, allergies, aches, brain fog, insomnia, libido issues, and more all typically appear - essentially the body communicating distress from excessive toxic friction.

Sometimes genetic predisposition focuses the damage predominately into one weak area. Other times toxins randomly disrupt a vulnerable tissue. But universally bioaccumulation threatens normal functioning *if not continually cleared out.*

This provides definitive rationale for prioritizing detoxification through programs like The New Cleanse - sickness is not typically bad luck but rather bad pollution! We bear responsibility to limit contamination instead of waiting for diagnoses.

The next chapter will overview specifically how our cleansing organs operate to fight back against toxins when supported appropriately...

Chapter 3: The Role of the Liver, Kidneys, Colon and Skin in Natural Detoxification

In the last two chapters, we defined the staggering array of toxins jeopardizing human health along with the primary modes of contamination and storage. With toxicity as a prime driver of nearly all chronic illness, the imperative for detoxification comes clearly into focus.

Fortunately, our bodies innately develop sophisticated systems to identify and eradicate threats - generally categorized into:

1) Transforming - Altering chemical structure of toxins to reduce harm

2) Eliminating - Removing toxic agents from the body

3) Healing - Repairing damage inflicted by exposure

In this chapter, we will closely examine the key organs tasked with executing these jobs - predominantly the liver, kidneys, skin, and colon. Appreciating their innate capabilities when operating optimally casts the mechanics of our cleanse protocol in a sensible light. We simply aim to facilitate what the body intrinsically does - when not obstructed.

Understanding natural detox mechanisms also underscores why more aggressive interventions like chelation require oversight. Broad spectrum healing rests first on supporting inborn pathways.

The Liver - Commander of Detoxification

As the largest visceral organ weighing about 3 pounds, the liver's epic responsibilities include:

- Metabolizing fats, carbs, proteins into usable energy

- Manufacturing essential compounds like albumin, fibrinogen, cholesterol

- Processing nutrients from digestion into bioavailable forms

- Storing key vitamins, minerals, glucose to maintain homeostasis

- Regulating blood composition for fluid balance

- Detoxifying a wide range of toxins

In fact, the liver neutralizes over 200 billion foreign substances daily! No wonder liver dysfunction strongly associates with countless chronic diseases.

The innate detoxification capabilities of the liver center around filtering blood coming from the digestive tract before circulation to body tissues. Specialized liver cells called **hepatocytes** use a two-phase enzymatic process to achieve chemical breakdown.

Phase 1 deploys alkaline compounds to create reactive sites on toxin molecules via oxidation, reduction or other transformations. This prepares the substrate for breakdown but initially generates reactive intermediates still requiring further processing.

Here common reactions include:

- Cytochrome P450 enzyme family oxidizing toxins

- Flavin monooxygenase system adding or removing oxygen groups

If phase 1 enzymes become overwhelmed however from toxin overload or nutrient depletion, excess intermediates spill over causing free radical damage.

Assuming proper nutritional status supporting adequate phase 1 activity, **Phase 2** then utilizes acquired reactive sites to conjugate transformed compounds for excretion.

This facilitates coupling with carrier molecules including:

- Glutathione - sulphur containing peptide

- Sulfate - involved in hormone and neurotransmitter metabolism

- Glycine - amino acid assisting bile formation

- Glucuronic acid - carbohydrate from glucose aiding water solubility for kidney removal

- Methyl groups - basic components preparatory for urine excretion

The tandem phase 1 and 2 sequence allows for impressive chemical versatility in metabolizing toxins. Dietary plant compounds like indoles and polyphenols additionally boost endogenous antioxidants to bolster the cascade.

However, when insufficient protein intake or vitamin deficiencies impair production, accumulating reactive intermediates create inflammation + tissue damage.

This intricacy underscores why both activating drainage pathways AND providing vital cofactors proves essential to reinforce systemic cleansing rigorously.

The Gut - Gatekeeper to Detox Flow

While the liver commands central detoxification authority, no organ better demonstrates interconnection with the total body ecosystem than the gut. In fact Hippocrates himself proclaimed over 2500 years ago that "all disease begins in the gut."

Modern research continues validating digestive tract health as the epicenter of overall wellness or illness. We each house over 100 trillion gut bacteria dictating inflammation cascades, nutrient absorption, hormone regulation, immune function plus direct impacts on digestion and detox organ efficiency.

Specifically for drainage pathways, the gastrointestinal system heavily influences natural cleansing processes through:

1) Microbiome Toxicity - Dysbiosis and intestinal permeability issues allow more toxin absorption from the gut into circulation rather than timely elimination.

Common culprits include weakened mucosal lining from chronic stress, antibiotics use or recurrent infections permitting larger macromolecules to infiltrate blood flow.

Simultaneously, certain opportunistic bacteria species release waste products like lipopolysaccharides (LPS) triggering widespread inflammatory consequences.

2) Bile Flow Regulation - Bile produced by the liver concentrates metabolic byproducts and toxins before excretion through feces. However bile also facilitates fat breakdown and nutrient absorption when recycled back to the liver.

If thickened bile or gallstones inhibit adequate bile flow, toxins and excess hormones get reabsorbed through enterohepatic recycling disrupting endocrine pathways.

3) Prebiotic Fiber Fermentation - Beneficial flora thrive on non-digestible fibers from plants which convert into short chain fatty acids. These compounds help reduce intestinal permeability and also support detoxification mechanisms.

Without adequate vegetables in the diet, good bacteria cannot derive enough sustenance to proliferate protectively.

This interrelationship emphasizes why rebalancing gut ecology using probiotics, antimicrobial botanicals and prebiotic fibers AS a centerpiece of our cleanse proves so essential for decongesting natural drainage channels.

The Kidneys - Underrated Detox Dynamos

The kidneys perform extraordinary filtration of the nearly 200 liters of blood traversing them daily. While largely recognized for fluid regulation and electrolyte balance, the kidneys also serve as a key defense node against toxicity.

Renal tissue actively secretes toxins into urine flow while conserving nutritive compounds for reuse in a brilliant display of selective permeability. Supporting kidney performance and urinary flow as part of our cleanse can liberate a significant element of the total toxic burden.

Key elimination roles include:

1) **Toxin Filtration** - Each day kidneys process about 200 quarts of fluid filtering out soluble waste, debris and chemicals for excretion. Toxins not cleared sufficiently accumulate causing nephron damage.

2) **Toxic Metabolite Excretion** - Conjugated hepatic byproducts from phase 2 detoxification undergo active transport into kidney tubules to exit via urine. Blood urea created from protein metabolism also drains here.

3) **Acid-Base Regulation** - Kidneys help modulate systemic pH by selectively reabsorbing or secreting acid or alkaline salts. This provides a buffered environment for cells to function optimally.

4) **Blood Pressure Control** - By regulating sodium levels and body water content, the kidneys indirectly stabilize blood pressure within healthy range.

This broad functionality emphasizes why kidney care through cleansing routines proves invaluable. Herbs like dandelion, nettle, cranberry plus ample hydration all bolster integrity of this filtration workhorse.

The Skin - Underappreciated Channel

While rarely perceived as a detox organ compared to the visceral heavyweights, ample evidence demonstrates how crucial healthy sweating patterns contribute to cleansing capacity.

With over 2 million sweat glands distributed across our skin enlisted to manage core temperature and homeostasis, the multifaceted usefulness of perspiration gets overlooked.

Toxic heavy metals like mercury, aluminum and lead all appear in concentrations up to 100 times higher in sweat compared to blood serum. This hints at the skin's capabilities.

Supporting robust perspiratory flow as in our sauna-based cleanse interventions meaningfully reduces systemic toxin stores over time. This millennia-old healing tradition persists for good reason!

Working Together as a System

Mapping the properties of each individual detox organ helps strategize support. However, we must avoid siloed thinking. Physiology fundamentally integrates all components as a unified process.

The liver synthesizes carrier molecules to shuttle waste from cellular cleanup to kidney filtration for exiting through urine. Meanwhile biotransformed compounds dump into the GI tract for removal through bile or feces. Skin perfusion regulates heat and fluid balance enabling stable organ function.

When alignment falters, toxicity accumulates damaging all areas of this ecosystem. Fortunately, the reverse also holds true - when we nourish and sustain detox potential, the whole-body terrain benefits. Our cells thrive when the rivers of metabolic waste flow smoothly. This defines the guiding intent of our New Cleanse.

In later sections we will address exactly how to energize cleansing systems through food, nutrients, herbs, sweat, stress relief and more. But first we must set the stage by quantifying the baseline toxic load needing rehabilitation...

Part II: Preparing for Your Detox

With a firm grounding now in the types of toxins jeopardizing health along with how the body innately counters those threats, we progress to the therapeutic protocols that actively facilitate cleansing processes.

Specifically in Part II, we will address critical preparation steps laying the foundation before undertaking a structured detoxification program like The New Cleanse. Rushing hastily into intensive interventions without proper precautions risks unnecessary discomfort, inadequate results or even harm.

Instead taking time to understand your current toxin exposures, establish the right detox mindset, and begin transitioning dietary habits proves integral for safe, effective cleansing.

Key preparation topics include:

Assessing Toxic Load - Surveying sources of recent toxin exposure through environmental and lifestyle audit questionnaires. This approximates the overall purification work needed.

Establishing Intentions - Clarifying personal motivations, goals and desired outcomes helps anchor the cleansing period with more conscious purpose and clarity.

Shifting Mindset - Adopting paradigm beliefs that support detox mechanisms proves invaluable. We address common limiting beliefs that sabotage progress.

Reducing Toxic Exposure - Minimizing contaminant intake from food, water and products lowers the baseline toxin burden entering the body. This pre-emptively lightens the detox workload.

Transitioning Diet - Gradual changes over 2 weeks to remove inflammatory foods, emphasize liver supporting nutrients and improve digestion. This gives time to adjust while priming detox organs.

Adequately preparing mentally, emotionally and physically proves crucial for tolerating temporary detox reactions smoothly. It also allows cleaner to derive maximal benefits from the full program. Rushing this foundation frequently causes people to quit prematurely.

Let's begin surveying your current lifestyle and environmental factors to approximate the overall toxic load requiring drainage...

Chapter 4: Determining Your Current Toxic Load with Assessments

Now that we have outlined the main categories of toxins and their common effects, the next step involves assessing your personal level of exposure. Quantifying exposure sources and symptoms provides key data points to customize your detox protocol accordingly.

This chapter will overview the primary questionnaires and evaluations to complete before undertaking a structured cleanse. The insights uncovered help approximate the overall toxic burden accumulated as well approximate key organs and systems needing focused support.

Common reasons for undergoing periodic cleansing include:

- Chronic diseases or stubborn symptoms not resolving

- Reaching a plateau in your current wellness program

- Overcoming an acute illness or major stressor more quickly

- Enhancing energy, appearance and cognition as prevention

- Pre-conception cleansing to reduce fertility issues and birth defects

- Slowing aging and boosting lifespan by reducing inflammation

But without quantifying factors contributing to your toxic load, applying broad spectrum detox therapies remains generic. Personalizing dietary modifications, supplemental support, detailing follow up lab testing etc allows us to strategically target inefficiencies for superior benefits.

Initial Toxicity Questionnaires

I recommend beginning assessment with the following surveys to reflect on exposure history:

1. Environmental Factors Audit

Catalogue prior occupational or hobby chemical hazards. Detail out residence locations, home age and renovations implicating solvents, paints, glues, particle board etc. Analyze deliberate and incidental proximity to industrial factories, incinerators, waste sites, airports exposing you to heavy metals and pollution run off.

Recall residences with mold, renovation dust exposure or sick building syndrome. Contemplate regular routes traversing high traffic pollution corridors. These environmental insults accumulate over years or decades stalling vitality.

2. Lifestyle Toxicity Audit

Self audit use of conventional body care products with parabens, phthalates, sodium laureth sulfate, artificial fragrance and colors. Review regular consumption of canned food and drinks in plastic or BPA lined containers allowing chemical leaching.

Consider exposure to food additives, flavor enhancers and sugary snacks that burden liver detox pathways and alter gut permeability. Reflect on medication history - antibiotics, antacids, steroids, anticholinergics. Even OTC pain pills like acetaminophen tax detox organs.

Catalog any metal dental work or implants interacting with tissues. Did you receive the standard aluminum loaded vaccine schedule or yearly flu shots with mercury? All of these low dose exposures contribute incrementally to bioaccumulation over months and years.

Finally calculate total hours of electronic device usage - especially wifi enabled laptops and phones - emitting DNA destabilizing non-native EMFs at unprecedented levels today. Few recognize this invisible radiation as an emerging toxin source in the modern world.

Reviewing all lifestyle factors through this lens highlights surprising vectors we tolerate daily that inhibit natural detox mechanisms when compounded. The silver lining exists in now consciously moderating these once you possess knowledge of subtle harms.

3. Symptom Severity Tracker

Beyond quantifying environmental and behavioral exposure sources, assessing symptom severity provides tangible feedback on how your energy, fitness and wellbeing change in response to interventions.

Tracking variability also helps gauge emerging detoxification reactions versus actual illness when undertaking an intensive cleanse program.

I recommend downloading a multi symptom health tracker app or using a simple 1 to 10 rating scale to monitor issues including:

- Low energy/fatigue

- Joint/muscle aches

- Headaches

- Brain fog/poor concentration

- Skin irritation

- Digestion complaints - bloating, cramps, loose stools

- Poor sleep quality

- Low libido

- Emotional volatility/mood swings

- Sinus congestion

- Yeast infections

Logging symptoms episodically before, during and after cleansing provides an invaluable progress barometer. Analyzing spike triggers also informs individual detox pathways needing special support.

Layering these questionnaires provides initial insight into sources, degree and clinical manifestations of toxin exposure. However we can still deepen investigation through functional lab testing next...

Functional Lab Assessments

While no perfect measure exists for quantifying true "body burden", specialized lab panels help approximate toxic infiltration and also identify key vulnerabilities:

1. Toxic Element Profile - Urine or hair analysis tests offering metal screening including arsenic, aluminum, cadmium, lead, mercury, nickel, uranium. This approximates bioaccumulation.

2. Organic Toxins Screen - Panels checking blood serum or urine for solvents, plasticizers, pesticides, PCBs, fire retardants and other environmental chemical residues.

3. Microbiome Analysis - DNA stool sample establishing proportions of beneficial flora strains versus opportunistic organisms. Indicates permeability/inflammation issues.

4. Nutrient Status - Blood, urine or hair testing detailing nutrient cofactors involved with liver detox reactions like B vitamins, zinc, selenium, magnesium, molybdenum etc. Deficiencies severely impact pathways.

5. Liver Enzyme Profile - Markers like AST, ALT and bilirubin quantify liver stress. Optimal ranges facilitate smooth biotransformation.

6. Lipid Panel - Provides breakdown of cholesterol fractions, triglycerides and particle sizes related to fatty liver disease interfering with toxin clearance.

These targeted analyses provide functional interpretation of internal body ecology compared to standard blood panels reporting rudimentary reference ranges. They serve as both helpful baseline benchmarks along with post cleanse re-evaluation of areas improved.

Genetic Considerations

A detailed discussion of genetic polymorphisms affecting detox enzyme functioning extends beyond our current scope. However recognizing common variations that potentially reduce natural toxin processing capacity proves useful when interpreting severity of symptoms.

For example, deficits in glutathione production or glycine conjugation pathways hamper ability to manage free radical cascades and chemical byproducts. Those with weakened sulfuration genes convert environmental toxins and neurotransmitters less efficiently.

Compromised Nrf2 activation interferes with switching on cellular defense genes normally countering oxidative damage. Impairments along detox superhighways mean harmful intermediates get created without adequate neutralization.

Testing companies like 23andMe provide reports detailing SNPs affecting particular cytoprotective genes. Understanding vulnerabilities here helps personalize nutritional cofactors to support clearance pathways. Those with certain defects often report dramatic benefits from rigorous cleanse regimens that sideline genetic handicaps.

While condensing complex topics inherently loses some nuance, hopefully this overview of evaluating toxic load and drainage capacity provides context to begin customizing your detox journey. The next two chapters offer additional customization through clarifying inner purpose and optimizing mindset...

Chapter 5: Setting Intentions and Establishing the Right Mindset

With the sprawling sources of toxicity quantified from the assessment questionnaires and proposed lab panels, this next phase of preparation focuses inward. Specifically cultivating supportive mental and emotional habits that empower cleansing mechanisms to operate smoothly.

Detoxification resides as much an internal biochemical process as an external set of practices. The two domains dynamically impact each other - either obstructing or enabling flow. *Our interpretations, beliefs and intentions surrounding cleansing exert incredible influence on tangible physiological outcomes.*

Hence consciously priming your internal landscape, rather than just passively undergoing protocols, makes all the difference between a mildly beneficial cleanse versus a profoundly regenerative experience.

In this chapter we will cover:

- Clarifying motivations and defining desired outcomes

- Identifying limiting beliefs that restrict detox mechanisms

- Establishing empowered beliefs aligned with the body's innate capabilities

- Helpful mindfulness techniques and visualizations

While subtle initially, adjusting mental patterns liberates cleansing potential equal to or beyond physical interventions alone. Combining both sparks alchemy.

Articulating Intentions

Before diving into a strict cleanse program, I encourage spending quality time reflecting on your underlying motivations and specific goals. Is the driving impetus primarily prevention to maintain vigor as you age? Or are you seeking symptom relief for a nagging health condition?

Get clear on intended benefits you wish to actualize from undertaking this intensive process. Write them down. The outcomes can span concrete physical targets like losing weight or getting off medications to more esoteric spiritual objectives involving personal growth and self realization.

Also examine any secondary gains or hidden motivations like wanting validation or using the cleanse to punish yourself. Becoming aware of unconscious emotional entanglements allows them to unwind before hijacking progress.

This simple introspective clarity aligns your navigation through sometimes uncomfortable cleansing reactions. With a defined destination encoded, you understand temporary symptoms reflect navigating ebb and flow currents towards renewed stability. Without firmly etched goals and incentives however, mild discomforts easily overwhelm conviction straying you off course.

Revisit your defined intentions frequently, especially when challenges arise. This north star helps override reactive sabotaging impulses to quit prematurely. You expand self mastery through consciously harnessing motivation despite hurdles. Maintaining solutions focus makes weathering the unpredictability easier.

Limiting Beliefs

Equally if not more important than crystallizing positive aspirations exists identifying ingrained assumptions potentially obstructing you. Commonly these themes include:

Fear of toxins - "My past exposure already permanently damaged my health. It feels pointless trying to correct now."

Lack of self efficacy - "My genetics make me helpless. Cleansing seems too difficult for me manage."

Underestimating body's wisdom - "Supports are needed forever because my body cannot regulate itself."

Failing to honor signals - "Detox symptoms mean something is wrong with the cleanse protocol rather than my body finding balance."

Seeking perfection - "If I cannot follow the plan perfectly or have specific symptoms, then there is no point continuing."

Do any self sabotaging stories resonate as familiar refrain held unconsciously? Shining light on these parasitic memes diminishes their control over behaviors that derail cleansing efforts.

We must nurture more empowered perspectives aligned with the incredible self healing capacities encoded into physiology. The key involves getting ego out of the way so body wisdom can come forward. *When provided proper inputs, our cells innately know how to recalibrate and thrive.*

From this lens, guidance like structured cleanse protocols simply removes obstacles so self repair programming can smoothly run. The power always resides inside you. An effective cleanse merely liberates this latent wisdom to manifest without internal interference.

Helpful Mindsets

Here are some supportive mental frameworks to invoke instead that facilitate detox mechanism efficiency:

Temporary discomfort is positive feedback - Allow symptoms to guide troubleshooting rather than discouraging progress. They indicate areas needing attention.

My body knows how to heal and rebalance - Trust symptoms represent innate intelligence re calibrating systems, rather than something breaking.

Small consistent progress adds up - Stay focused day to day without fixating on the big picture. Cumulative benefits build momentum.

I lovingly give my organs extra support - Imagine nutrients, herbs and therapies nurturing natural detoxification capacity.

My vitality continually expands - Assume positive changes will unfold with persistence through the process.

Reinforcing these affirmative attitudes sets the stage for a regenerative experience. They unlock maximal benefits from the physical detox protocols engaged. Again, intentions exert incredible influence - for better or worse.

Helpful Visualization Techniques

Imagery provides another portal for priming mindset if helpful. Visualizing nutrients and anti-inflammatory compounds bathing tissues trains emotional receptivity for physical interventions. Some simple 5-minute meditations include:

1. Breathe slowly while envisioning oxygen cleansing every cell. Oxygen represents the ultimate nourishment carrying life force energy.

2. Imagine each sip of broth washing GI lining removing debris so mucosa renews. Think of the recipe ingredients reversing inflammation.

3. Picture the sauna heat helping open elimination channels for toxins to drain out while micronutrients enter.

Use creative license to invent helpful metaphors that emotionally resonate and reinforce trusting body detoxification abilities. The placebo impact stretches far beyond inert sugar pills into the consciousness brought to all healing modalities. Spend time nurturing how you relate to cleansing practices for amplified effectiveness.

When paired with proven physical support strategies outlined later, applying intentional awareness practices leverages maximum synergy helping accelerate results. Too often overlooked, establishing the right mindset gifts leverage no supplemental formula alone can impart...

Chapter 6: Pre-Cleanse Diet - Reducing Toxic Exposure Over 2 Weeks

Now that we have set firm intentions and adopted an empowered mindset, we complete preparation by reducing inbound toxin exposure through dietary upgrades.

Tuning the instrument before playing allows musicians to hit notes cleanly. Similarly optimizing digestion capacity before intensifying detoxification proves foundational to handling increased drainage smoothly.

This chapter details stepwise dietary guidelines for a 2-week pre-cleanse period to:

1) Minimize inflammatory foods interfering with detox pathways

2) Increase key liver supporting nutrients to bolster drainage mechanisms

3) Improve bowel eliminations to reduce reabsorption of toxins

4) Hydrate tissues and prime kidney filtration capacity

5) Allow time for palate changes and obtaining new ingredients

The gradual incremental upgrades lessen discomfort when transitioning to the full cleanse regimen later. Quick abrupt shifts provoke harsh reactions. Gentle acclimation invites more sustainable change.

Many new ingredients get introduced over the coming pages. Do not attempt adopting everything simultaneously. Take it stepwise at your own pace. Consistency over time brings the biggest net gains.

Week 1 Diet Upgrades

Eliminate:

- Sugar, high fructose corn syrup, artificial sweeteners

- Fried foods and trans fats

- Conventional dairy products

- Excess caffeine intake over 200mg daily

- Soda, energy drinks, alcohol

Reduce Intake Of:

- Conventional red meat: aim for once weekly or swap for buffalo, lamb, venison

- Gluten grains: avoid excessive wheat, barley - swap for heritage grains like rice, buckwheat, millet, corn

- Factory farmed eggs: purchase pasture raised whenever possible

Increase:

- Filtered water intake + herbal detox teas - 2-3 liters daily

- Organic vegetables + low sugar fruits - 1 pound daily

- Clean high-quality fats + oils - olives, avocado, nuts/seeds, ghee, extra virgin olive/coconut oil

- Fermented foods - unsweetened yogurt, kefir, kvass, kimchi, sauerkraut

- Herbs/spices - turmeric, garlic, ginger, cayenne, cinammon

- High fiber intake > 35 grams daily - vegetables, berries, flax, chia

This initial wave of elimination provides straight forward swaps lowering dietary contributions to inflammation and toxic burden.

Plentiful vegetables encourage improved bowel motility to limit enterohepatic recirculation of toxins and hormone metabolites.

Herbs aid liver enzyme function while fermented foods start rebalancing digestive flora. Simply curbing sugar excess lowers a major stressor to metabolic pathways.

These foundational upgrades offer the lowest hanging fruit to bolster energy levels and mood heading into the cleanse while avoiding overwhelm. Now in week 2 we deepen changes.

Week 2 Diet Upgrades

Eliminate:

- Factory farmed meat + eggs

- Processed grains/breads

- Refined seed oils: canola, grapeseed, sunflower, corn, soybean etc

- Raw cruciferous veggies: kale, broccoli, cauliflower, cabbage etc

- Microwaved foods in plastic containers

Reduce/Limit:

- Beans/legumes: encourage 2-3 meatless days per week

- Starchy carbs

- Nightshade's veggies if personally reactive - tomatoes, peppers, potatoes

- Fruit and natural sweeteners

Increase:

- Organic pastured meat 1-2 weekly - beef, poultry, pork

- Wild caught low mercury fish + seafood 2-3 weekly - salmon, sardines, cod

- More fat intake at meals

- Rainbow spectrum vegetables, leafy greens daily

- Probiotic and fiber rich traditional foods - pickled items, bone broth, organ meats

These more advanced changes aim to curb common gut irritants while flooding your diet with mineral rich ingredients that support natural detoxification processes. The cumulative benefits prepare your body to handle elevated toxin drainage during the intense 3 week protocol ahead.

While seemingly strict on paper initially, embracing traditional food wisdom reveals how many cultures around the world adopt cleansing diets inherently through cultural staples. Humans thrived for millennia eating nourishing recipes that detox by default. We have only deviated into poor health recently.

Supplemental Support Over 2 Weeks

Beyond upgrading dietary foundations over this transitional period, adding supplemental support primes detox organ function.

I suggest starting a daily regimen based on personal needs including:

Liver Herbs: Milk thistle, turmeric, schisandra berry, artichoke leaf

Probiotics: Multi strain high potency formulas - minimum 30 billion CFUs

Prebiotic Fiber: Baobab, acacia, arabinogalactans and inulin sources

Bowel Motility Agents: Magnesium, vitamin C, triphala, dandelion root

Antimicrobials: Oregano oil, berberine, caprylic acid, undecylenic acid zinc

Micronutrient Cofactors: B complex, zinc picolinate 25mg, methylated B12

These represent basic interventions easily incorporated into daily habits that enhance natural organ function, microbial balance, hydration and transit supporting a smooth transition when intensifying cleansing efforts.

The ultimate goal aims for metabolically efficient digestion through this preparation period. Optimizing GI terrain then allows cleaner foods and targeted botanicals to elevate drainage capacity coordinating the liver, gut lining, microbiome, kidneys and lymphatics.

As new chapters detail the structured cleanse chronology, having already cultivated foundational dietary and supplemental habits makes adopting further protocols far easier. Too often people attempt Layering all changes simultaneously then struggle with compliance and quickly rebound to old habits that sabotage success.

Instead visualize the pre cleanse period like training for an athletic event. You gradually build capacity so that the real workload ahead gets handled smoothly having eliminated easily correctable deficiencies beforehand. The next section examines common symptoms during this ramp up window.

Interpreting Transitional Reactions

As the body accommodates cleaner fuels, increased water intake, targeted supplementation and reduced intake of allergenic foods/chemicals, temporary symptoms may arise termed **"detoxification reactions"**.

These generally represent a positive sign of shifting terrain, not problems to suppress. However navigating them without context often deters people incorrectly. Understanding common transient symptoms empowers persistence through temporary turbulence towards improved baseline functioning.

1. Fatigue - Carb and sugar cravings subside as cells wean off glycolysis metabolism. Until mitochondrial density improves, lower energy prevails. Supplementing B vitamins, magnesium and ubiquinol converts this quickly.

2. Aches - Anti inflammatory foods reduce pain signals. Toxins releasing also trigger inflammatory responses transiently. Supporting elimination channels helps decrease duration.

3. Digestive complaints - Loose stools, constipation, bloating and pain reflect gut flora rebalancing. Stay hydrated and supplement probiotics until it stabilizes.

4. Skin Breakouts - Liver pathways route toxins out alternative exits. Allowing temporary irritation prevents deeper reabsorption. Don't pick, nurture elimination.

The intensity and duration of symptoms provides key data revealing overall toxicity load and deficits needing correction. Tracking variability also shows you when terrain restores equilibrium as symptoms decline over weeks.

In most cases, symptoms represent noise not needing suppression since they indicate healing underway. But don't hesitate consulting a functional medicine practitioner if you have concerns or high discomfort.

With foundational elements now established through dietary upgrades, intentional mindset shifts and targeted supplement support, you complete preparation for intensive cleansing protocols ahead...

The next section covers the structured chronology of The New Cleanse 21 day system.

Part III: The New Cleanse 21-Day Detox Program

Having laid the appropriate dietary, supplemental and mindset foundations in preparation, we now launch into the core protocols defining the 21-day New Cleanse detoxification program.

Part III provides a day-by-day breakdown of structured interventions across three 7-day phases designed specifically to:

1. Initiate cellular cleanup processes through fasting mechanisms

2. Flush debris from interstitial spaces between cells

3. Open elimination channels supporting toxin removal

4. Flood the body with micronutrients as cofactors for biotransformation enzyme reactions

5. Rebalance gut ecology and nourish mucosa to heal permeability

6. Stimulate lymph flow to direct wastes towards kidney filtration

The coordinated detox wave moves sequentially through organs and tissues facilitating powerful upstream and downstream effects through phase progression.

Toxin removal extending to the intracellular level allows genuine healing and regeneration to commence. This enables lasting benefits unlike compartmentalized "juice cleanses" lacking comprehensive support.

The layered protocols interweave multiple traditions of cleansing including:

- Intermittent fasting for cellular autophagy

- Gut healing nutrients and botanicals from Ayurveda

- Liver supporting compounds from Traditional Chinese Medicine

- Lymphatic techniques from European biological medicine

- Kidney drainage remedies from naturopathy

- Targeted supplementation from functional nutrition

The harmonious fusion empowers this program to operate on multiple fronts simultaneously. No single isolated modality alone matches this dynamic physiology rooted synergy.

Let's overview the arc of progression across the complete cleanse journey before detailing specifics day to day...

Chapter 7: Overview of the 3-Phase Detox Program

Having equipped you with all the requisite knowledge surrounding toxins and cleansing mechanisms along with supportive preparation steps, we finally arrive at the structured protocol section itself - *the heartbeat of our 21 day New Detox journey.*

This opening chapter surveys the overarching flow across phases so you understand the teleology before we delve into the minutiae day-to-day. Grasping the cascading logic of progression allows navigation of temporary detox discomforts with motivated clarity rather than just blind rigidity.

Let's explore the terrain...

Cleanse Flow Overview

The program navigates three 7-day phases tuned to serve specific physiological purposes:

Phase 1 - Cleanse - We first gently enter a fasted, introspective state to unlock cellular cleanup processes and initiate toxicity drainage at the roots.

Phase 2 - Restore - With debris now displaced from the extracellular environment, we emphasize nourishment and glandular repair to foster recuperation.

Phase 3 - Revitalize - Having cleared obstructions and rebuilt energetic reserves, we finale by sealing the fortified terrain with protective practices for sustainable optimization.

Week-to-Week Objectives

Week 1 - Cleanse

Goal: Commence cellular detox through intermittent fasting, kidney support, lymph stimulation

Focus: Blood, interstitial fluids, intracellular spaces

Week 2 - Restore

Goal: Nourish and heal detox organs + gut lining to consolidate gains

Focus: Digestion, microbiome, liver, gallbladder, kidneys, endocrine system

Week 3 - Revitalize

Goal: Fortify longstanding benefits through alkaline minerals, antioxidants and lifestyle upgrades

Focus: Vitamin/mineral status, pH balancing, stress resilience, prevention

You can observe the cascading interconnection as phases build sequentially. Toxin displacement starts from the capillary level before replenishing those now liberated cellular niches with upgraded nutrition and targeted antioxidants.

We stimulate drainage channels through intermittent fasting, heat therapy, manual techniques and selected botanicals to maintain output without congestion. Gut healing and rebalancing digestive flora helps ensure enclosed toxins get liberated into eliminative routes rather than reabsorbed ongoingly.

As with any flow dynamic, some degree of cyclical backflow between organs persists through each week. However the predominant emphasis shifts upstream to downstream in a coordinated progressive fashion.

Now that we have oriented the master blueprint, let's overview core techniques deployed through the journey to actualize the protocol objectives...

Key Detox Agents Across Phases

Liquid Fasting - Structured intermittent fasting with alkaline fluids lets gut rest while activating autophagy cellular cleanup.

Phytonutrient Concentrates - Cold pressed juices, micronized greens, berries and aloe nourish interstitial spaces.

Glandular Extracts - Raw organ and tissue extracts supply bioactive compounds supporting weakened organs.

Probiotics and Digestive Enzymes - Improve nutrient absorption and rebalance microbiome strains.

Antimicrobials - Yeast/parasite cleansing opens eliminative routes for drainage.

Liver Support Nutrients - Lipotropics thin bile while antioxidants spur biotransformation reactions.

Lymphatic Techniques - Rebounding, massage and sauna improve lymph circulation removing wastes.

Botanical Chelators - Specific plant compounds help usher out heavy metals through urine or bile.

Kidney Flushing - Alkaline hydration with botanical diuretics prevents renal stagnation allowing exited toxins to flow out smoothly.

Lifestyle Upgrades - Dialing in nutritive foods, efficient exercise, community and nature contact seals the integrative healing process.

Mastering the ability to weave these detox agents expertly provides the art form separating formulaic cleansing programs from transformational experiential journeys into renewed vitality.

We leverage the multifaceted techniques in coordinated waves - moving from intracellular spaces outward to tissue planes then evacuation through emunctories - to enable genuine physiological cleansing absent in simplistic methodologies.

Now that you have glimpsed the bird's eye view of progression, we will break down exactly what each day entails from supplements to recipes to practices over the ensuing pages...

Chapter 8: Phase 1 - The 7 Day Cleanse

Having outlined the master flow across the full 21 days, we now dive into the daily details defining Phase 1 - our 7 day cleanse. This intensive period aims to:

- Initiate cellular detoxification via fasting mechanisms

- Dislodge toxicity from extracellular spaces and tissues

- Direct liberated toxins into eliminative channels

- Prevent mobilized wastes from getting reabsorbed

- Set the stage for strengthened nourishment absorption to come

We focus first on displacing debris as the highest initial priority. Creating vacant niches allows gentler Phase 2 nutrients to uptake optimally upon refeeding. Attempting substantial repair prematurely while occlusion remains risks feeding residual unwanted elements still embedded.

Hence, we emphasize lymph, blood and interstitial matrix drainage support through Phase 1 knowing we will replenish the relative depletion appropriately during Restore. Avoiding the indulgence of immediate gratification gifts exponentially more profundity.

Here are the key techniques deployed throughout the week to actualize those detox goals:

1. Structured Liquid Fasting - The core foundation arresting digestive workload involves abstaining from solid foods while hydrating with alkaline fluids allowing gut rest. Extended fasting elicits unique cleansing reactions we leverage purposefully during the cleanse.

2. Micro Nutrient Delivery - Cold pressed juices, micronized greens, aloe, berries and whole food concentrates nourish tissues without demanding full digestion. We emphasize antioxidants to balance free radical fluxes.

3. Lymphatic Stimulation - Rebounding, massage and sauna improve flow through extracellular channels transporting liberated cellular debris towards liver and kidneys for processing.

4. Digestive Repair - Removing irritants allows intestinal lining to heal while antimicrobial botanicals rebalance compromised flora reducing inflammatory byproducts in circulation.

Now let's explore what exactly each day looks like through the cleanse...

Day 1 Objectives

The opening day goals involve:

- Allow digestive focus to move upstream through liquid nourishment to initiate cellular repair

- Introduce foundational filtered fluids, electrolytes, trace minerals

- Get clarity on intended cleanse journey purpose

Daily Protocol

7am: 32 oz lemon water with electrolytes upon awakening

8am: Green juice or plant based smoothie

10am: Clear vegetable broth with collagen powder

12pm: 25-30 oz structured water

3pm: Green juice or berry phytonutrient smoothie

6pm: Clear miso broth with coriander, fennel, cardamom and ginger

9pm: Detox tea - dandelion, milk thistle root, burdock root

We focus on hydrating well to support kidney filtration fluid dynamics as lymph stimulation later will increase drainage. Light broth-based meals give the gut extended rest while providing minerals and amino acids.

Ample organic electrolytes help prevent fatigue, cravings and headaches. We emphasize greens and berries for antioxidants balancing free radical bursts. Journal to capture any detox sensations arising as healing commences.

Wellness techniques:

- Oil pull with coconut oil upon awakening

- Dry skin brushing before shower

- Fun dance workout movements to favorite music tracks

- Light yoga flow if desired

- Review prepared intentions clarity

Day 2 Objectives

We progress detox momentum by:

- Increasing lymph flow to direct toxins into circulatory routes

- Supporting kidney filtration capacity with botanicals

- Providing micronutrients to match elimination efforts

Daily Protocol

Same structured fasting fluid regimen as Day 1

Additional Nutrients:

- Digestive enzymes with meals
- 1 Tbsp Aloe juice

- Probiotic capsule before bed

- Nettle and dandelion glycerite extract midday

Wellness Techniques:

- Rebounder workout for 10 minutes

- Take digestive bitters before vegetable broth meals

- Calming Epsom salt foot soak at night

The emphasis on dodder seed, nettle leaf, corn silk, horsetail, dandelion introduces mild natural diuretics increasing urine output without taxing kidneys. This prevents mobilized debris from settling back into tissues.

Aloe vera compounds further support intestinal repair and microbiome balance easing transport through membranes. Enjoy restorative leisure or community time as energy permits in the evening.

Day 3 Objectives

Expanding upon drainage momentum, we:

- Intensify lymphatic flow through increased rebounding

- Further support kidney function with marshmallow root

- Lean into any detox reactions for informational feedback

Daily Protocol

Same structured fasting fluids as prior days

Additional Support:

- 30 minutes rebounding split morning and afternoon

- Marshmallow root and cinnamon tea

- 2 tsp diatomaceous earth before bed

- Multimineral supplement with potassium broth

Wellness Techniques:

- Oil massage scalp and lymph nodes before showering

- Alternate hot and cold showers for 2 minutes at end

- Handstands against wall to invert gravity draining lymphatics

- Add Epsom salts or peroxide to bathwater for absorption

- Journal reflection on sensations

Pushing movement, circulation and breathing a bit more aerobically turns up cellular furnace activity dislodging oxidative debris into fluids. Supporting flow ensures transit. Diatomaceous earth binds to toxins entering digestion from bile and guts assisting elimination through bowel movements.

Monitor energy levels closely avoiding fatigue by bumping electrolytes and fluids if demanded. However, embrace the inward focus as purification accelerates. Discomfort guides learning.

Day 4 Objectives

Midway through the cleanse emphasizes continuity moving metrics:

- Maintain integrity of fast for cellular cleanup

- Improve fatty acid status to support liver phase 1 detox

- Introduce antimicrobial botanicals for microbial balancing

Daily Protocol

Same structured fasting fluids as prior days

Additional Support:

- Digestive enzymes with veggies

- 2 Tbsp cod liver oil

- Oregano leaf tincture before meals

- Magnesium broth or bath soak

Wellness Techniques

- Dry skin brushing exfoliation

- Foam roll tight neglected muscle groups

- Alternate hot and cold shower 2 minutes

- Breath of fire breathing 5 minutes

- Take leisurely walk outside barefoot

Cod liver oil supplies bioavailable vitamin A for liver phase 1 reactions along with anti-inflammatory eicosatetraenoic and docosahexaenoic acids assisting cellular debris clearance. Oregano, garlic, ginger bitters support microbiome rebalancing efforts.

Grounding to the earth's surface releases static buildup from inflamed tissues. Avoid overtiring with activity today keeping eliminative focus. Traffic sometimes increases as terrain shifts - this is positive. Look for reproducibility of symptoms correlating to intervals between drainage aids like rebounding, massaging lymph nodes, sauna or Epsom salt baths. Track trends through journaling.

Day 5 Objectives

The later cleanse days feature continuity cranking channels supporting heightened filtration capacity:

- Maintain integrity of fast for cellular cleanup

- Introduce colon cleanse for improved eliminations

- Support kidney health with increased herbs and fluids

Daily Protocol

Same structured fasting fluids as prior days

Additional Support:

- Intestinal cleanse formula AM and PM
- 1 tsp each: nettle, corn silk, marshmallow root
- Ginger, garlic lemon tea
- 1 Tbsp cod liver oil

Wellness Techniques:

- Skin brushing before rebounding
- Yoga squat holds to strengthen elimination
- Alternate hot and cold shower 3 minutes
- Lymph massage down each limb towards heart
- Relax in non-EMF nature settings

The triphala based intestinal cleanser improves bowel elimination binding to metabolites, plastics, hormone debris and bile sludge escorting excretion without griping. Continuity flushing kidneys maintains open exits so debris doesn't reabsorb elsewhere.

Light resistance training online or home workouts boost metabolism and circulation if energy permits. Otherwise nurture restorative practices. Observe mindset for resistance or fears arising to highlight areas needing compassion. Symptoms still provide cleansing feedback.

Day 6 Objectives

The penultimate cleanse day keeps consistency rolling while assessing energy floors:

- Maintain integrity of liquid only nourishment
- De-sludge bile flow to support exiting toxins
- Further boost glutathione production

Daily Protocol

Same structured fasting fluids as prior days

Additional Support:

- Ox bile supplement before meals

- Liposomal glutathione spray 3x daily

- Lemon water with cayenne and fulvic throughout day

Wellness Techniques:

- Practice alternate nostril breathing

- Take detoxifying Epsom salt bath

- Gentle yoga for improved lymph and blood flow

- Skin brush towards heart before bed

- Early sleep for neural restoration

Ox bile salts thin thicker bile improving liver dump flow into intestines for final cleanup. Liposomal glutathione drives key antioxidant production to temper inflammatory fallout as debris exits. We coast the downhill finish line staying consistent.

Check in on original cleansing intentions. Notice areas of tangibility through the process so far - sensation, mentation, sleep, elimination, skin, breath changes? Much recalibration still percolates under the hood preparing for our Restore phase...

Day 7 Objectives

The closing cleanse day intends integration looking forward:

- Close fast gently transitioning digestion

- Introduce light broth and vegetable meals

- Support sustainable kidney filtration

- Inventory systems still needing attention

Daily Protocol

7am: Gentle fruit and greens smoothie

10am: Clear vegetable broth with protein boost

1pm: Large green salad with hemp seeds, sprouts, dressing

4pm: Golden milk tea with collagen powder

7pm: Coconut cauliflower rice stir fry with ginger/lemongrass

Additional Support:

- Kidney support tonic tea

- Triphala before bed

- Magnesium transdermal spray

Wellness Techniques:

- Breath focus throughout day

- Light yoga for grounding

- Alternate hot and cold shower

- Dry skin brush towards heart

- Sauna session followed by cold plunge

We break the fast with easier to digest smoothies and soups to welcome back peristalsis motions before adding fiber. Light whole foods provide balanced nourishment as we enter Restore phase appetite. Tapering botanical support prevents backsliding.

Reflect on improvements through the week - energy, bowel movements, sinuses, bloating, pain levels, seasonal allergies etc. Also make notes on areas still needing attention moving forward. Phenomenal alchemy percolates under the hood!

Chapter 9: Phase 2 - The 7 Day Restore

With immense cellular revitalization catalyzed paving cleaner terrain, we progress to Phase 2 emphasizing uptake of nutritive elements to fortify regeneration.

Where the Cleanse phase focused on excavating dysfunction, these Restore days now infuse upgraded materials sealing the structural repairs underway.

Our goals this week involve:

1. Nourishing the detox organs and glandular system

2. Repairing intestinal lining integrity to improve assimilation

3. Rebalancing microbiome strains for sustainable immunity

4. Flooding tissues with minerals, cofactors and phytonutrients

5. Providing building blocks to strengthen structural proteins

We still facilitate some degree of elimination support while attenuating intensity. However the orientation shifts upstream from the capillary lymphatic level during the cleanse towards functional organs and digestion during restore.

Relaxing the detox jets slightly allows fuller absorption of nourishing inputs rather than having nutrients diverted towards processing waste outflows. We strategically feed the vacuum created through week 1 evacuation.

Let's survey how the daily protocols actualize those goals...

Day 8 Objectives

As we coast off the cleanse momentum, first day emphasis includes:

- Improving protein assimilation efficiency

- Repairing small intestinal barrier integrity

- Continuing microbiome rebalancing efforts

- Inventorying organs still needing TLC

Daily Protocol

7am: Aloe protein smoothie with coconut milk

10am: Beetroot and fennel liver supportive soup

1pm: Stomach healing seaweed salad

3pm: Adrenal glandular extract

6pm: Thyme and sage antibacterial chicken

9pm: Soothing gut restore tea

Additional Support:

- Digestive enzymes with meals

- Marshmallow and slippery elm supplements

- Prebiotic fiber rich foods

- Ox bile before largest meal

Wellness techniques:

- Oil massage abdomen and feet

- Gentle twisting yoga poses

- Walking meditation outdoors

- Alternate hot and cold shower

Emphasizing easily digestible amino acids with limited inflammation generating foods, we prop stomach healing using demulcent and mucilaginous plant foods. Our intention focuses on sealing intestinal permeability to prevent pickup of pathogens or food antigens increasing immune workload.

Gently continuing lymphatic and circulation support prevents backsliding. Check on original symptoms - is the terrain continuing to improve? What organs feel most nourished by the cleanse? Which still need attention?

Day 9 Objectives

Expanding digestive repair efforts, we:

- Improve hydrochloric acid levels for protein breakdown

- Include bitter teas and enzymes stimulating bile flow

- Fortify mineral stores chelated for bioavailability

Daily Protocol

7am: Warming aduki bean apple porridge

10am: Mineral rich bone broth soup

1pm: Bitter dandelion and chamomile tea

3pm: Zinc and magnesium supplements

6pm: Ginger miso glazed cod with vegetable stir fry

9pm: Gentle triphala nightly cleanse

Additional Support:

- Digestive bitters before larger meals

- Ox bile supplements as needed

- Continue marshmallow root 1 tsp

Wellness Techniques:

- Belly massage along colon in clockwise motion

- Try castor oil pack over liver area

- Light rebounding or yoga for circulation

- Alternate hot and cold shower

Increasing natural bitters from dandelion, gentian, ginger and digestive enzymes bolsters our own HCL acid production to improve protein breakdown from clean foods. We emphasize mineral rich bone broths and whole food concentrates to correct deficits before introducing denser proteins next phase.

Gentle yoga twists encourage lymphatic and bile flow. Moving posture flows keep tissues healthy. Check on original symptoms again - are more modalities improving?

Day 10 Objectives

Nearing the halfway mark this renovation phase, we:

- Expand variety of nourishing proteins

- Emphasize antioxidant rich vegetables

- Support ongoing kidney and bladder health

Daily Protocol

7am: Buckwheat crepe stacked with nuts, seeds and fruit

10am: Free form vegetable soup with wild rice

1pm: Cranberry peach kidney tea

3pm: Curried tempeh over quinoa

6pm: Pistachio crusted salmon with herb salad

9pm: Chamomile and passionflower tonic

Additional Support:

- Digestive enzymes as needed

- Nettle leaf infusions

- NAC antioxidant support

Wellness Techniques:

- Self lymphatic drainage massage

- Moderate hiking or biking outdoors

- Alternate hot and cold shower

- Yoga for improved circulation

- Sauna session

Expanding diet diversity beyond elimination phase increases satisfaction while avoiding gut irritants. Antioxidant rich deeply hued veggies flood tissues with phytonutrients and polyphenols missing during the cleanse week. Staying activeOUTDOORS resets circadian biology and grounds nervous system.

Day 11 Objectives

As microbiome balance normalizes, we:

- Up nutrition density further with nuts/seeds/sprouted grains

- Introduce fermented items repopulating probiotics

- Shift focus from drainage towards assimilation

Daily Protocol

7am: Chia seed berry probiotic yogurt

10am: Carrot and beet kvass

1pm: Pineapple crisp salad with sprouted chickpeas

3pm: Pumpkin seed pesto linguine pasta

6pm: Red lentil coconut curry

9pm: Golden turmeric nightly tonic

Additional Support:

- Enzymes as needed

- Slippery elm before meals

- Marshmallow and licorice tea

Wellness Techniques:

- Nasal saline wash

- Tennis, basketball or jogging

- Stretching hip flexors, chest and shoulders

- Dry skin brush towards heart

Incorporating fermented foods once bacterial terrain normalizes provides natural probiotics to reseed gut colonies. The prebiotics in nutrient garnishes feed beneficial flora stabilizing renewal.

We emphasize antioxidant anti-inflammatory spices that improve flavors while enhancing cellular defense. Light activity energizes musculoskeletal fitness. How are original symptoms this week compared to day 1?

Day 12 Objectives

As restore phase enters closing stretch, we:

- Expand palate richness with spices, marinades, dressings

- Maintain alkaline minerals from broths and veggies

- Prepare the terrain for increased protein next phase

Daily Protocol

7am: Savory cumin egg frittata

10am: Mung bean spinach soup

1pm: Pineapple mango gazpacho

3pm: Zucchini curry coconut wraps

6pm: Rosemary lamb chops with wild rice

9pm: Chamomile passionflower relax tonic

Additional Support:

- Enzymes with dense meals

- Nettle infusions for minerals

- Aloe juice support

Wellness Techniques:

- Tennis or gentle weights routine

- Alternate hot and cold shower

- Dry skin brush towards heart

- Fun dance session to music

Culinary herbs make minerals and phytochemicals more bioavailable while stimulating digestive secretions. Their antibacterial compounds also hasten intestinal lining repair we initiated day 1. Continue pushing circulation with activity for sustained results.

Day 13 Objectives

In our final Restore surge before the Revitalize anchor phase, we:

- Introduce nutritive glandular concentrates

- Provide liver support if needed

- Inventory remaining areas needing improvement

Daily Protocol

7am: Scrambled eggs with thyroid, liver pâté

10am: Golden milk turmeric tea

1pm: Spinach and liver salad

3pm: Aloe vera juice smoothie

6pm: Lamb kidneys with marrow gravy, sweet potato

9pm: Liver/gallbladder flush tea

Additional Support:

- Digestive enzymes

- Milk thistle, turmeric, selenium

- Continue probiotics

Wellness Techniques:

- Light weights and resistance bands

- Skin brushing towards heart before shower

- Relaxing music session breathing

We tap into the profound regenerative nutrition within organ meats and glandulars to nourish weakened tissue matrices. Continuing antioxidant support aids ongoing liver phase 1 and 2 functioning protecting DNA. Bitters before meals keep smooth bile flow.

Reflect again on tangible cleanse improvements so far - energy, cravings, allergies, pain levels, seasonal sensitivities etc. What modalities served you best? Which still need troubleshooting? Our final week seals the integrated terrain...

Chapter 10: Phase 3 - Revitalize (7 Days)

After completing the first two phases of cleansing and restoration, you are now ready for the third and final phase - revitalization. This 7-day phase will help rebuild healthy cells, recharge your energy levels, and revitalize your body and mind.

Rebuilding Healthy Cells

The first focus of the Revitalize phase is **rebuilding healthy new cells**. Your cells play a vital role in detoxification, energy production, immune function, and overall health. But after years of exposure to toxins and processed foods, many of your body's cells are likely worn out or functioning poorly.

That is why the Revitalize diet emphasizes the most **nutrient-dense whole foods**. These superfoods provide high levels of antioxidants, phytonutrients, vitamins, and minerals to restore optimal cellular health:

- Brightly colored fruits and vegetables - greens, berries, citrus fruits

- Nutritious grains and legumes - quinoa, brown rice, lentils

- Healing herbs and spices - turmeric, ginger, cinnamon

- Healthy fats and oils - avocado, olive oil, coconut oil

- Clean proteins - wild salmon, grass-fed meats

Focus on incorporating more of these healing foods into your diet over the next 7 days. For quick and easy meal ideas, turn to the recipes in **Part VI**. Dishes like the Strawberry Spinach Salad, Immune Boost Soup, and Citrus Salmon Bowl provide targeted nutrition to rejuvenate your cells.

In addition to diet changes, certain **lifestyle habits** support healthy cell regeneration:

- Hydration - Drink half your body weight in oz of clean water

- Exercise - Practice both HIIT workouts and gentle movement like yoga

- Sleep - Get at least 8 hours of sleep nightly

- Stress relief - Practice meditation, breathwork, or forest bathing

By combining whole foods, targeted nutrients, and supportive lifestyle behaviors, your cells will renew and rebuild themselves stronger than ever.

Recharging Your Energy

The second important focus of the 7-day Revitalize phase is **recharging your energy levels**. Cleansing can often leave you feeling a bit drained physically and mentally in the short term. So it is vital to refuel with natural energy boosters as your body recovers.

The Revitalize diet incorporates many foods that deliver **sustained energy**:

- Fruit - For an instant boost from natural fructose

- Leafy greens - Magnesium prevents fatigue and weakness

- Healthy fats - Omega-3s reduce inflammation causing fatigue

- Protein - Amino acids provide steady energy and stamina

- Spices - Ginger, cinnamon improve circulation and energy

In addition to a nutrient-packed diet, adopting certain practices helps **optimize energy absorption**:

- Proper food combining - Pair carbs + fat or protein + veggies

- Smaller, frequent meals - 5-6 smaller meals rather than 3 large

- Timed eating - Eat carbs in mornings or pre-workout

- Mindful eating - Relaxed pace, chew thoroughly

Finally, there are several **adaptogens and supplements** recommended during Phase 3 to boost energy:

- Cordyceps - Increases ATP cellular energy

- Rhodiola - Helps body adapt to stressors

- Iron - Improves blood oxygen transport

- B Complex - Supports mitochondrial energy creation

As you provide your body the proper building blocks and support, your natural energy levels will steadily climb back up by the end of the 7 days.

Revitalizing Your Body and Mind

The last goal of the phase is to renew your sense of **physical health and mental wellbeing** - your body and mind. Cleansing aims to revitalize you in a holistic manner, from the cells up.

To fully rejuvenate during this phase, engage in practices that are recharging, enjoyable, and aligned with your intentions:

Physical Revitalization

- **Movement** that you love - yoga, dance, hiking, swimming

- Bodywork therapies - massage, acupuncture, sound baths

- Nature immersion - beach, mountain, forest experiences

- Home spa rituals - Epsom salt baths, dry brushing

Mental/Emotional Revitalization:

- **Creativity** - art, music, writing

- **Presence** - meditation, breathwork

- **Inspiration** - uplifting podcasts, books

- **Connections** - quality time with loved ones

This is your time to nourish body, mind and spirit with healing foods, activities, places or people that bring you joy and renewal of energy.

Continuing Forward after the Detox

As you reach the completion of the 21-day detox, you should feel a renewed sense of health, vibrancy and clarity. But the work does not stop here!

Be sure to read:

- **Chapter 16** for post-cleanse recommendations

- **Chapter 17** for maintaining clean living

- The **Conclusion** for final tips

The ultimate goal is to carry forward the healthy diet and lifestyle habits you formed over the past 3 weeks. With commitment to these positive changes, you will continue cleansing, restoring and revitalizing your body for months and years to come.

Now take this fresh start and run with it! Keep learning, growing and exploring what else helps you feel healthy and energized every day.

Part IV: Supporting Your Body's Natural Detox Capabilities

As you now understand, your body has an incredible inborn detoxification system, centered around key organs like the liver, kidneys, skin and gut. When operating optimally, this network of detox organs and pathways effectively filters out toxins so they can exit your body safely.

However, when your detox organs become overloaded or inefficient due to toxicity, poor diet, chronic stress or other factors, your natural cleansing processes break down. Toxins then accumulate within your body, leading to a range of negative mental, physical or emotional health effects.

The good news is you have the power to restart and support your body's detox abilities so they work efficiently again! Making strategic diet and lifestyle changes gives your detox organs exactly what they need to heal and cleanse at full capacity once more.

That is why Part IV provides comprehensive, holistic guidance to enhance your body's detox capabilities from the inside out. The next 4 chapters will cover:

- **Chapter 11:** The New Cleanse Diet - principles and food guide for nourishing detox

- **Chapter 12:** Tips to detox your home, work and life environments

- **Chapter 13:** 10-minute daily cleansing routines to stimulate detox pathways

- **Chapter 14:** Choosing the best detox supplements to further support organ health

With the combination of healing whole foods, reduced toxic exposures, active cleansing rituals and selective supplements, you give your body exactly what it craves to restart natural detox processes.

Rather than extreme or depriving cleanses, **the New Cleanse approach is gentle yet effective at promoting the body's innate intelligence**. It works *with* your natural systems, not against them. When aligned properly, your body knows exactly what to do - cleanse itself optimally and return to balance effortlessly!

So, get ready to fully support all your major detox pathways and organs over the next 4 chapters. By becoming an active participant in your body's self-cleaning mission, you allow deep cleansing and revitalization to unfold - safely, efficiently and completely naturally.

Chapter 11: The New Cleanse Diet Principles and Food Guide

What you eat each day has a direct impact on your body's ability to detoxify and cleanse itself. Adopting strategic diet changes gives your detox organs like the liver and kidneys exactly what they crave to function optimally and flush out accumulated toxins with ease.

That is why food lies at the very foundation of the New Cleanse detox approach. First, this chapter will overview the guiding **principles** for what makes up an ideal detox diet. Then, it will provide a detailed **food guide** outlining the optimal whole foods to emphasize and avoid during your cleanse.

5 Principles of The New Cleanse Diet

There are 5 core principles that characterize the ideal diet to support natural detoxification:

1. Organic, Whole Foods

Focus your diet on unprocessed, organic, whole plant and animal foods. Not only are these less toxic, but they provide a plethora of cleansing nutrients, enzymes and fibers your organs need.

2. Nutrient Density

Emphasize foods with a high density of detox-promoting vitamins, minerals, antioxidants and phytonutrients per bite. These nutrients directly facilitate your main detox pathways.

3. Alkalinity

Prioritize alkaline foods over acidic. Alkaline environments allow your cells and detox organs to function optimally and facilitate elimination of toxins.

4. Plant Diversity

Eat a colorful variety of plants and botanicals. Diverse plant compounds stimulate cleansing enzymes and provide fiber to support elimination.

5. Balance Blood Sugar

Choose low glycemic foods that won't spike blood sugar. Steady energy prevents cravings, overeating and fat storage - which burden detox organs.

Using these 5 simple guidelines for what to eat each day allows your body to cleanse itself naturally and effectively.

The New Cleanse Diet - Food Guide

Here is a detailed guide on the optimal foods to focus on (or avoid) when cleansing:

Fruits and Vegetables

As the foundation of any cleanse diet, these should make up 50-70% of daily intake. The phytonutrients, enzymes, minerals, and fiber directly enhance detox organ and pathway function while alkalinizing the body.

Eat an abundance of:

- All leafy greens

- Crucifers: broccoli, kale, arugula, Brussels sprouts, cabbage

- Deeply coloredproduce: berries, beets, tomatoes, carrots, peppers, citrus

- Raw fruitsand veggies for enzymes

- Sea vegetables: nori, kelp, wakame

Limit or avoid:

- Starchy veggies: corn, peas, white potato, sweet potato

- Higher sugar fruits: pineapple, mango, grapes, banana

- Canned, frozen, or juice - only fresh!

Clean Proteins

Moderate protein intake provides amino acids to produce cleansing enzymes and glutathione while helping stabilize blood sugar. Get 15-25% of calories from clean, organic sources.

Excellent sources:

- Wild fish: salmon, sardines

- Shellfish: oysters, mussels

- Grass-fed beef or bison

- Pasture-raised poultry

- Organic eggs

- Plant-based proteins: beans, lentils, natto

Avoid:

- Factory farmed meat

- Soy protein isolates

- Whey protein isolates

Healthy Fats

Omega fatty acids aid liver health while coconut oil supports gut detox. Get 20-30% of calories from primarily plant-based fats that balance blood sugar.

Beneficial fats:

- Avocado

- Extra virgin olive oil

- Flax and chia seeds

- Hemp, walnut and sesame oils

- Coconut oil or butter

Limit:

- Butter or ghee

- Non-organic dairy fat

- Conventional nuts or oils

Cleansing Carbs

The right carbs provide antioxidants along with fiber to sweep toxins out through bile and bowel movements. Stick to 25-30% of diet from clean complex carbs.

Eat often:

- All sprouted or fermented grains

- Quinoa

- Brown rice

- Sweet potato

- Winter squash

- Beans and lentils

Greatly limit:

- Gluten grains

- Corn

- White rice

- White potato

Healing Herbs and Spices

Herbs like cilantro, garlic and milk thistle support liver function while ginger improves digestion and detox. Use spices liberally to flavor foods over salt.

Key herbs and spices for detox:

- Turmeric

- Ginger

- Garlic

- Onion

- Milk thistle

- Dandelion

- Cilantro

- Cinnamon

- Cayenne

- Apple cider vinegar

That covers the optimal whole foods to emphasize for cleansing while limiting toxic exposures. Use this guide as your blueprint for dietary changes that allow your body's natural intelligence to cleanse and recover effectively. Refer to the recipe section for delicious ways to implement these healing foods.

Chapter 12: Tips for Home and Life Detox

While diet plays a central role, creating a clean living environment is equally important when undergoing a detox. Toxins perpetually enter your body through not just food, but also air, water, household products and medicines.

That is why in addition to an internal cellular cleanse, you must also purge toxins from your external home, work and life environments. This dual approach allows you to reduce toxic exposures so your detox pathways can direct all their efforts internally rather than constantly battling new chemicals.

Here are tips to detoxify your living spaces, possessions, and lifestyle habits in support of your internal cleanse.

Cleaning Products

Conventional cleaning supplies and laundry detergents contain a cocktail of harsh irritants, chemicals and artificial fragrances that get absorbed through your skin or fumes that you breathe in.

Replace with non-toxic, eco-friendly alternatives:

- All-natural dish and laundry soaps

- Vinegar, baking soda, hydrogen peroxide

- Essential oil cleaners - lemon, tea tree oil

- Microfiber cloths over paper towels

- Castile bar soap for hands/body

- Natural loofahs and brushes vs plastic

Personal Care Products

Toxins easily enter the bloodstream through the highly absorptive skin, scalp, and mucous membranes. Reduce this exposure by swapping body care products for organic, pure options:

Skin and body:

- Plant oils - coconut, olive, almond

- Shea butter

- Castile bar soap

- Mineral based make-up

Hair:

- Shampoo - organic essential oils

- Apple cider rinses

- Sea salt spray

Oral:

- Tooth powder

- Tongue scraper

- Activated charcoal

Household:

- Beeswax food wraps vs plastic

- Natural loofahs and brushes

Home and Office

Indoor living areas often harbor hidden toxins in furniture, electronics, building materials and home goods. Purge and upgrade items adding unnecessary toxicity:

- Replace Teflon, plastic food containers with glass

- Swap synthetic furniture/carpets for natural fibers

- Install HEPA filters, salt lamps, air purifying plants

- Open windows regularly for fresh outdoor air

- Use hardwire internet connection not WiFi

- Minimal electronics in bedrooms

Filtered Water

Tap water contains remnants of chlorine, fluoride, pharmaceutical drugs, microplastics and heavy metals. Install high quality home filters for drinking, cooking, bathing and cleaning to avoid absorbing these through skin or digestive system.

Options like reverse osmosis, carbon block, ceramic and sediment filters all drastically reduce contaminants. Shower filters also cut down on absorption through the lungs and skin.

Organic Matresses and Bedding

Since you spend a third of life asleep, make sure your resting area is toxin-free. Most mattresses and bedding contain flame retardants, formaldehyde and other chemicals that accumulate in your body as you sweat and shed skin cells overnight.

Replace with:

- Organic cotton, wool bedding

- Natural latex, coconut coir or bamboo mattresses

- Low EMF emitting space

Medications and Supplements

Conventional OTC meds and prescription drugs add an intense toxic load through the liver and kidneys to filter. Minimize intake of these unless absolutely necessary during cleanses.

Also audit supplements for fillers, flow agents or preservatives common in capsules and tablets. Seek out high quality professional brands using only pure ingredients.

Relax and Destress

Psychological and emotional stress releases cortisol, adrenaline, cytokines and other inflammatory chemicals that burden detox pathways, especially the liver and gut.

Make time each day to actively relax through:

- Yoga, breathwork

- Forest bathing

- Massage, float therapy

- Nature sounds/music

- Laughing, hugged, napping

A clean-living environment and lifestyle habits relieve the toxic load on your body's natural detox systems dramatically. This allows your organs to focus cleansing inward rather than constantly defending against chemical inputs from outside.

Chapter 13: 10-Minute Daily Cleansing Routines

In addition to a cleanse diet and reduced toxin exposures, it is important to actively stimulate and support detoxification pathways regularly.

This chapter provides 10-minute routines you can engage in daily while cleansing to further enhance elimination functions. Like giving pipes a flush, these quick rituals essentially "take out the trash" by flushing waste out through key exit routes.

Practice each routine first thing in the morning on an empty stomach whenever possible. Or split them up throughout the day if needed. These complementary cleansing tactics boost results from your diet and lifestyle changes.

Stimulate Lymphatic Drainage

The lymphatic system serves as the body's drainage system with nodes and vessels that collect cellular waste and filter toxins. However, unlike blood flow it lacks a pump and relies on physical movement to drain.

Spend 5 minutes performing lymphatic stimulation:

- **Dry skin brushing** - Brush skin towards heart

- **Rebounding** - Jump on mini trampoline

- **Lymphatic yoga** - Cat/cow, twists, inversion poses

- **Deep breaths** - Deep inhales stimulate flow

This movement "wrings" the lymphatic system to push toxins towards exit points.

Hydrate and Flush with Lemon Water

One of the simplest yet effective ways to flush both the liver and kidneys is drinking plenty of fluids, especially mineral rich or citrus-infused water.

Drink a 16 oz glass of room temperature lemon water first thing when you wake up. The bioactive citric acid helps stimulate bile and urine production to flush waste out quicker through stool and urine. Aim to finish within 5 minutes.

Follow with another 16 oz of plain water 15-30 minutes before meals to aid digestion. Proper hydration keeps elimination routes fluid and flowing.

Dry Brush Skin

As your body's largest organ, the skin plays a key role in waste elimination through sweating and shedding dead skin cells. Exfoliate and stimulate sweat glands and lymph drainage with 5 minutes of dry brushing before showering.

Use a natural bristle brush and brush the skin in circular motions towards the heart. Focus on areas that don't often get direct exfoliation like back, sides and back of legs.

Finish with an invigorating cold rinse to close pores.

Oil Pulling for Oral Detox

Oil pulling draws toxins out of the blood and lymphatic fluid in the mouth before they can be reabsorbed. Swish around 1 Tbsp coconut oil in the mouth for 5-10 minutes then spit out. Coconut oil has antibacterial properties and also removes plaque.

For deeper oral cleansing, use a natural bristle toothbrush with baking soda and mineral tooth powder to scrub tongue and teeth. Rinse with an antiseptic essential oil mouthwash. Reducing oral bacteria and toxins prevents reabsorption.

Dry Skin Brushing

As your body's largest organ, the skin plays a key role in waste elimination through sweating and shedding dead skin cells. Exfoliate and stimulate sweat glands and lymph drainage with 5 minutes of dry brushing before showering.

Use a natural bristle brush and brush the skin in circular motions towards the heart. Focus on areas that don't often get direct exfoliation like back, sides and back of legs.

Finish with an invigorating cold rinse to close pores.

Digestive Tonics and Enzymes

Boosting digestion and bowel movements eliminates toxins the body has filtered out into bile or stool. These tonics stimulate digestion, reduce gas and bloating, and promote healthy gut flora:

Bitters tonic - 2 droppersful bitters in 2 oz water

ACV - 1 Tbsp apple cider vinegar in 4 oz water

Probiotic - capsule before meals

Digestive enzymes - capsule with heavier meals

Spending just 5 minutes on these tonics before larger meals maintains regularity and speeds transit time through the digestive tract.

Actively Sweat

Our skin plays a key role in detoxification and sweating is one of its waste elimination processes. Engage in 10 minutes of exercise or activity that makes you actively sweat such as rebounding, running, biking, dancing or sauna.

Follow any vigorous sweating episode by quickly rinsing off without soap then hydrating to replace fluids and minerals lost through perspiration.

Nasal Cleansing

The nasal passages offer a quick absorption route straight to the bloodstream as well as directly filtering air we breathe. Reduce environmental exposures while removing mucus accumulations by rinsing sinuses.

Use a Neti pot, bulb syringe or nasal aspirator to run pH balanced saline solution through nasal cavity and out other nostril. Saline wash keeps membranes hydrated and flushed.

Skin Cleansing

The skin eliminates toxins through sweating and shedding dead skin cells from the epidermis. Exfoliate buildup and stimulate lymph drainage with 5 minutes of dry brushing before showering.

Use a natural bristle brush and brush the skin in circular motions towards the heart. Focus on areas that don't often get direct exfoliation like back, sides and back of legs.

Finish with an invigorating cold rinse to close pores.

Practice these quick but highly effective rituals daily alongside your detox diet, supplements and lifestyle adjustments. Actively supporting better elimination through key pathways gives your body the nudge it needs to deepen cleansing effects dramatically. Be consistent for 10 minutes daily and feel the cumulative benefits!

Chapter 14: Choosing the Right Detox Supplements and Herbs

While whole foods, movement and lifestyle practices form the foundation of effective cleansing, certain supplements can provide targeted support.

The right herbs, nutrients, glandulars or botanicals enhance specific detox pathways or organ function. Think of them like helpers that improve flow, speed eliminations or protect organs as increased toxins get processed.

However, with the hugely expansive supplement industry, quality and efficacy varies greatly. This chapter will overview the safest, most research-backed detox supporters to consider adding to amplify your cleanse.

Top Detox Organ Supports

Certain supplements directly aid, nourish or tone the key detox organs to improve their filtration abilities:

Liver Support

Milk Thistle- The premier liver herb, it boosts production of glutathione, the body's master detox antioxidant, while protecting liver cells. Take 175 mg, 2-3 times daily.

NAC - N-Acetyl Cysteine is a powerful antioxidant that raises glutathione levels. Take 500-600 mg daily on an empty stomach.

Beetroot or Dandelion Root - These bitters stimulate bile flow to improve fat digestion and elimination through stool.

Kidney Support

Cranberry Extract - Prevents bacteria adherence in urinary tract and increases urine flow to flush kidneys. Take 500 mg daily.

Marshmallow Root - Soothes urinary tissues irritated by toxins passing through. Take 2-4 grams powdered in tea or capsules.

Digestive Support

GI Detox - Binder supplements like activated charcoal, clay, pea fiber or psyllium husk help absorb and eliminate toxins, preventing reabsorption into bloodstream.

Probiotics - Support healthy gut flora, which aid digestion and protect intestinal barrier function. Take 25-50 billion CFU, twice daily.

This organ system support gives your natural filtration systems an added boost to work more efficiently during cleansing periods.

Detoxification Pathway Support

Other supplements fuel and enhance specific detox mechanisms in the body to flow better:

B Vitamins + C - Key cofactors in both Phase 1 and 2 liver detox that enable enzymes to convert and clear toxins out of body.

Turmeric - Boosts glutathione and bilirubin which neutralizes toxins in liver. Take 500-1000 mg curcumin daily.

Minerals - Himalayan salt, magnesium or potassium aid cellular detox function and electrolyte status for hydration.

Sulfur-Rich Foods - Crucifers, garlic, MSM and eggs provide sulfur to support both liver and skin detox pathways.

Providing vital co-nutrients for cellular pathways undergoing higher filtration volume prevents slow downs or back ups as toxin elimination increases.

Herbal System Tonics

Certain traditional herbs stimulate and strengthens the entire mind-body system to handle heightened detoxification and rebalancing effects:

Milk Thistle - repairs and protects liver cells overwhelmed by toxins

Burdock root - blood cleanser; increases circulation and lymphatic drainage

Dandelion - stimulates bile flow and enzyme production

Ginger - aids digestion and detox; reduces nausea

Reishi mushroom - adaptogen for mental clarity and immune defense

Peppermint - soothing GI tract; aids digestion

These broadly balancing botanicals make cleansing more comfortable and effective.

When to Use Supplements

Here are simple guidelines around timing and duration for detox supplements:

- Start organ system supports 1-2 weeks before a cleanse

- Take pathway cofactors just during active detox periods

- Use toning herbs as needed based on symptoms

- Only supplement for 2-4 weeks; give body breaks

Of course always read labels carefully for dosage guidelines based on the specific product and concentrations. And check with your doctor before supplementing if you have underlying health conditions or take any medications.

Used strategically, quality supplements reduce stress pathways may face trying to meet higher detox demands. This allows deeper cellular cleansing without overwhelmed key organs in the process.

Part V: Troubleshooting and Maintaining Detox

Congratulations, you have now completed the 21-day New Cleanse detox program! With commitment to the dietary protocols, lifestyle adjustments and cleansing rituals, you have guided your body through a deep yet gentle cellular detoxification.

However, the cleanse is only the first step in an ongoing purification process and journey towards optimal health. Remaining toxins stored in fat cells and organs will continue releasing over the next few weeks to months needing to get properly filtered out.

Therefore, the vital next phase is learning how to maintain detox momentum and adapt as symptoms or challenges arise. Rather than abruptly stopping all protocols, you must slowly transition into stabilizing the progress made.

That's why Part V offers troubleshooting guidance and post-cleanse recommendations to properly consolidate your gains. The next 3 chapters will cover:

- **Chapter 15** - What to do if unpleasant or unexpected symptoms appear

- **Chapter 16** – Post cleanse protocols to stick with over next month

- **Chapter 17** - Maintaining clean living habits long-term

While cleansing opens the exit routes for toxins to leave the body, it is equally important to support proper elimination following a cleanse while the body keeps detoxifying.

Implementing stabilizing protocols and responding effectively if cleansing reactions occur allows you to lock in positive changes through wise management. Supporting ongoing detoxification and adaptation ensures cellular purification continues unfolding to reach an even deeper level of balance and vibrant health.

Chapter 15: Troubleshooting Common Issues During a Detox

As toxins dislodge from cells and exit the body during a cleanse, you can experience some mild to moderate adjustment symptoms. These cleansing reactions are positive signs cellular detoxification is unfolding.

However, unpleasant symptoms can also indicate organs are overwhelmed trying to keep up with eliminating sudden toxin floods. Being able to troubleshoot common detox issues ensures proper support.

Here are effective solutions to the most frequent challenges:

Fatigue

As toxins exit energized mitochondria, reduced cellular output can translate into feeling drained, lethargic or weary. Support energy levels by:

- Check iron levels and supplement if indicated

- Increase mineral rich sea salt and electrolytes

- Add B complex for coenzyme support

- Reduce exercise intensity & get more rest

Once toxin release lightens, fatigue often passes within 1-2 days.

Headaches

Headaches arise due to dilated blood vessels or dehydration as kidneys filter more uric acid from cells. Relieve pain by:

- Drinking more lemon water - 64+ oz

- Taking magnesium citrate or glycinate

- Massaging pressure points

- Reducing toxin exposures

- Limiting fasts or caloric restrictions

Proper hydration and electrolyte balance typically alleviates headaches within several hours.

Changes in Bowel Habits

As the gut eliminates a heavier toxic load, stools can become loose, urgent, or more odorous. Or alternately, transient constipation may occur. Getting bowels back on track involves:

- Taking probiotic supplements

- Increasing magnesium-rich foods

- Massaging abdomen daily

- Trying digestive bitters or enzymes

- Avoiding gut irritants

Healthy gut flora and reduced transit time stabilizes bowels within 2-3 days typically. Monitor changes closely.

Skin Rashes or Break Outs

Skin eruptions result from lymphatic drainage systems overwhelmed trying to eliminate toxic backup too quickly. Support skin clearing by:

- Dry brushing to stimulate lymph flow

- Taking burdock root or nettle supplements

- Drinking organic celery juice

- Applying bentonite clay masks

- Avoiding reactive foods

Once drainage pathways catch up, rashes and breakouts heal after several days up to 2 weeks for more severe cases.

Flu-like Symptoms

Body aches, sore throat, stuffy nose or fever can manifest as circulating toxins trigger temporary inflammatory immune responses. Alleviate feelings by:

- Getting more rest

- Drinking pure electrolyte fluids

- Taking anti-inflammatory herbs like turmeric or ginger

- Applying essential oils - eucalyptus, peppermint, lavender

- Avoiding excessive exercise

Symptoms tend to pass within 48 hours once toxin circulation reduces.

Mood Changes or Anxiety

As toxins exit the nervous system, neurotransmitter changes can occur leading to feeling irritable, sad or worried. Stabilize mood by:

- Taking adaptogenic herbs like ashwagandha or reishi

- Avoiding toxin exposure from people, places or media

- Engaging parasympathetic relaxation response - yoga, meditation, nature

- Supplementing with magnesium, omegas, B vitamins

- Journaling feelings to process emotions

Releasing suppressed emotions allows moods to largely stabilize after several days to 2 weeks.

Other Potential Symptoms

- Sugar or junk food cravings as cells exit dysfunctional patterns

- Insomnia from excess cortisol or excited nervous system

- Muscle aches or weakness from electrolyte loss

- Low libido or lack of motivation from dopaminergic changes

Troubleshooting reactions using holistic supportive solutions allows detox symptoms to smoothly normalize. Be patient through any ups and downs, communicate with your practitioner, and tune into your body's needs. Cleansing and healing unfolds in layers and waves. With proper care through transitional moments, you will continue feeling better and better!

Chapter 16: Post-Cleanse Recommendations

Completing an intensive cellular detox is an important first step in your cleansing journey. However, removing accumulated toxins is just part of the equation. Equally important is sealing in your gains by supporting the body's transition back to balance.

This chapter outlines the top post-cleanse protocols to implement over the month following your detox program. These recommendations help stabilize improvements made and further deepen positive changes unfolding.

Follow the 80/20 Rule

Now that you've hit the reset button and achieved an inner baseline of health, adopt an 80/20 approach to your lifestyle habits.

- **80% of the time** strictly follow the cleanse diet principles, cleansing rituals, toxin avoidance habits and supportive practices. This sustains your renewed level of health.

- **20% of the time** incorporate modest indulgences if cravings arise or social events pop up. Having some leniency prevents an overly rigid or perfectionist mentality around eating and living "perfectly". Moderation and self-compassion is key.

This pareto principle allows you room to enjoy life's special moments without losing all your hard-earned success through a total rebound.

Slowly Taper Off Rigid Protocols

Just as you eased into the intense 21-day cleanse through a 2 week pre-cleanse preparation phase, tapering off slowly is equally important.

Abruptly stopping all detox protocols can shock your system after the body has acclimated to new rhythms and function patterns. Plus toxins continue releasing from tissues for weeks to months post-cleanse.

- **Week 1 Post-Cleanse:** Follow 75% of cleanse protocols at a reduced level

- **Week 2:** 50% detox protocols

- **Week 3:** 25% cleanse protocols

- **Week 4+:** Resume regular 80/20 lifestyle habits

Give your body ample time to readjust to balance as you slowly release strict regimens.

Continue Key Supplements

Certain supplements taken during your detox can continue providing targeted organ and pathway support 1-2 months post cleanse as well.

Liver & kidney supportive herbs help these filter organs that are still actively processing a heavier toxic load released from your cleanse. Milk thistle, NAC, marshmallow root and cranberries aid their resilience.

Minerals & electrolytes help stabilize cellular function, hydration and energy as your body repletes itself. Concentrate on magnesium, potassium and Himalayan sea salt.

Probiotics further enrich gut flora diversity aiding digestion, immunity and mental health.

Slowly ween off cleanse-specific supplements after 1-2 months though. Give your body breaks between intensive supplement regimes.

Address the Emotional and Spiritual

Alongside physical detoxification, mental, emotional and spiritual cleansing often occurs revealing old thought patterns, traumas or beliefs needing to be processed and released.

Make time for self-reflection through:

- **Journaling** - Write out thoughts, memories or emotions that surface

- **Talk therapy** - Discuss what arises with therapist or coach

- **Meditation** - Observe and let go of recurrent mental cycles

- **Creative expression** - Make art, music, poetry or dance with sensations

- **Time in nature** - Allow feelings to surface and move through you

Exploring inner realms revealed allows mental and spiritual aspects of your being to further cleanse and heal.

Transition Your Fitness Routine

During an intensive cellular detox, you limit intense exercise to conserve energy for healing. As you move forward, steadily resume workouts but avoid pushing too hard too fast.

- Week 1: Light walking, yoga, stretching

- Week 2: Moderate hiking, gentle bike rides, light weights

- Week 3: Advance as energy permits without overexertion

- Week 4: Steady state cardio, HIIT workouts

Honor days when your body says it simply needs more rest. Cleansed cells have higher energy output when truly restored.

Be patient transitioning fitness and monitor energy dips, fatigue, cravings or symptoms indicating you're overdoing activity. Your cleansed system knows exactly the right pace if you tune in.

Schedule Follow Up Assessments

3 months after completing your detox program, undergo follow up testing to tangibly assess improvements gained:

- **Dutch test** - adrenal, sex hormone, metabolism markers

- **Food sensitivity testing** - delayed IgG allergies

- **Digestive stool analysis** - gut/microbiome status

- **Blood work** - lipid panel, liver enzymes, vitamins

Use biomarkers to see which areas have reached optimal status and what may need further support through nutrition, herbs or lifestyle adjustments.

Be proud of tangible positive changes while still continuing work where progress is still needed! Healing happens through consistent layers.

Committing to smart transition protocols over the month following your detox locks in a radically improved baseline to build even greater health and wellness upon - in all areas of your life.

Chapter 17: Maintaining a Clean and Toxin-Free Lifestyle

Completing a detox program provides an incredible cleansing reboot and renewed sense of health. However the real question becomes: how do you maintain this higher level of wellbeing long-term without having to constantly detox?

The key is fully integrating the diet, lifestyle and environmental changes into your daily autopilot habits. This chapter gives practical tips to make clean, toxin-free living second nature.

Make the 80/20 Rule Your Default

In the last chapter, the short term 80/20 guideline was introduced for the month following a detox. As you settle back into everyday life, continue this pareto principle as your new normal lifestyle pattern:

- **80% of the time** - Follow all the cleanse diet principles for whole food meals, cleansing rituals, toxin avoidance habits and general healthy lifestyle protocols

- **20%** - Loosen up for special occasions, weekends or holidays

This sustainable balance allows you to maintain vibrancy and feel abundant in health without becoming overly fixated or restricted around food choices, activities or environmental exposures.

Make conscientious clean living the foundation while still enjoying yourself regularly!

Keep Elimination Channels Flowing

Now that your exit hatches for toxins are open post-cleanse, it's vital to keep waste flows moving consistently. Maintain daily rituals to promote elimination functions:

- Upon rising - Hot lemon water, dry brush skin, oil pulling

- Breakfast - Hydrate with electrolytes and mineral water

- Morning - Eliminate bowels first thing

- Post-workout - Cleanse skin through sweating/showering

- Evening - Take cleansing supplements before bed

Additionally, optimize digestion efficiency through consistent meals at the same times containing cleansing foods and combinations.

Keep pipes actively flushed!

Reduce Toxic Exposures

While we can never fully avoid toxins in the modern world, you can certainly minimize unnecessary exposures through smart lifestyle and consumer choices:

- Household & personal care products - Use only non-toxic, natural options

- Water filters - Install high quality filters on all drinking and shower sources

- Cleaning protocols - Open windows, use plants, consistently dust/vacuum

- Furniture & textiles - Replace synthetic materials with natural fibers

- Food storage & cooking - Swap all plastic for glass, ceramics, stainless steel

- Cosmetics & body products - Select pure, organic sources only

Making your home into a clean sanctuary protects your renewed level of health since this is where you spend most of life!

Adopt Cycles of Cleansing

Instead of waiting until you feel sluggish or sick to detox again, adopt intentional cycles of cleansing 2-4 times per year during seasonal changes.

This effectively "spring cleans" cellular gunk before it builds up enough to cause symptoms. Staying ahead of toxicity keeps your body humming!

Follow a simple protocol:

- **7-10 Days** - Follow strict detox diet and supplement protocols

- **1 Month After** - 80/20 eating with transition protocols

- **3 Months Later** - Get follow up testing to assess progress

Listen to the natural rhythms of nature's cycles guiding when your body needs a reboot.

Make Lifestyle Factors a Daily Priority

Don't abandon the positive lifestyle habits that bolstered your cleanse success! These daily practices protect cellular health and vibrant energy:

- **Exercise** you enjoy - Make movement non-negotiable

- **Stress relief** - Set boundaries, say no, relax intentionally

- **Nature immersion** - Forest bathing, beach, gardens

- **Sleep hygiene** - Unwind devices 1hr before bed, sleep by 10pm

- **Mindset habits** - Meditation, journaling, affinity spaces

By upholding supportive behaviors daily and not just during a detox, you extend the cleansed state achieved. Protect your temple!

- **Community & Accountability** - Surround yourself with people who support your healthy lifestyle goals rather than unknowingly sabotage them. Having friends or practitioners keeping you on track makes integration infinitely easier!

Following through with toxin avoidance, healthy protocols and balanced indulgences prevents needing to constantly detox. Listening and responding to your body's needs through cycles of cleansing and nourishment keeps you fully energized to embrace life's gifts!

Part VI: Recipes

One of the keys to sticking with the New Cleanse detox program is having delicious, nutritious foods to turn to that align with the diet protocols. Preparing tasty recipes centered around cleansing ingredients and combinations is essential.

That's why the final section of the book provides over 100 mouthwatering recipes specifically designed to:

- Give your body maximum phytonutrients and antioxidants

- Balance blood sugar levels and energy

- Hydrate and support eliminative organs

- Alkalize pH for optimal cellular function

- Provide anti-inflammatory, healing compounds

- Digest easily without causing gut distress

- Satisfy cravings through natural sweeteners and fats

With a medley of breakfasts, snacks, main entrees, sides and desserts, eating clean does not have to feel restrictive or bland! These recipes make it easy to get abundant flavor and satisfaction from nature's medicine foods.

All recipes indicate:

- Key detox ingredients

- Cleansing mechanisms and benefits

- Macronutrient & calorie totals

- Cook time and directions

- Modifications or serving suggestions

Additionally, each dish tags if it is particularly beneficial for:

- **Liver Support** - Beetroots, crucifers, turmeric, leafy greens

- **Kidney Aid** - Celery, berries, lemon, dandelion greens

- **Gut Soothing** - Fermented foods, broth, coconut oil

- **Anti-Inflammatory** - Wild fish, turmeric, ginger, berries

- **Energy Boost** - Adaptogens, clean carbs, avocado, apple

- **Nutrient Dense** - Dark leafy greens, sprouted grains, seeds

With this extensive recipe collection, the guesswork is taken out of preparing cleansing meals. Get ready to feel nourished and satisfied - not deprived! Let's get cooking...

Chapter 18: Smoothies

Smoothies make for the ultimate cleansing breakfasts or snacks. Blending together fiber-rich fruits and veggies maximizes nutrient absorption while requiring minimal digestion compared to eating whole produce.

You also pack a serious punch of antioxidants, phytonutrients, vitamins and minerals into one portable vessel. Just toss ingredients into your blender and you've got a custom elixir to boost cleansing and nourishment!

Play around with combinations based on what produce is freshest or seasons change. Swap out non-detox friendly smoothie staples like banana and milk for cleaner ingredients like zucchini or nut mylks.

Base Ingredients

Leafy Greens - Spinach, kale, swiss chard, romaine

Low Glycemic Fruit - Berries, green apple, grapefruit

Hydrating Liquid - Filtered water, coconut water, herbal tea

Healthy Fats - Avocado, coconut butter, hemp seeds

Cleansing Boosts - Lemon juice, ACV, fresh ginger, cinnamon

Berry Green Antioxidant Smoothie

- 2 cups spinach

- 1 cup mixed berries

- 1 green apple, chopped

- 1/2 avocado

- 1 Tbsp chia seeds

- 1 cup coconut water

- 1" ginger, peeled

- Blend until smooth.

Benefits – liver support, anti-inflammatory, nutrient dense

Per serving: 380 cal | 9g P | 50g C | 20g F | 12g fiber

Sweet Citrus Immunity Smoothie

- 2 cups chopped romaine

- 1 grapefruit, peeled

- 1 orange, peeled

- 1/2 cup pineapple

- 1 tsp turmeric

- 1 Tbsp aloe vera juice

- 1 cup filtered water

- Blend until smooth

Benefits – anti-inflammatory, kidney support

Per serving: 250 cal | 6g P | 58g C | 2.5g F | 7g fiber

Mint Choco Green Smoothie

- 2 cups baby spinach

- 2 Tbsp cacao powder

- 1 Tbsp almond butter

- 1 cup zucchini, chopped

- 1 cup coconut water

- 10 fresh mint leaves

- 1 tsp cinnamon

- 1 tsp vanilla extract

- Blend until smooth

Benefits – liver support, balances blood sugar

Per serving: 220 cal | 8g P | 36g C | 8g F | 7g fiber

Chapter 19: Salads and Dressings

Salads make the perfect cleansing lunch or dinner, packing a spectrum of phytonutrients, enzymes and fiber. Mix and match an array of organic, local greens and veggies topped with anti-inflammatory fats and herbs.

Salads also aid hydration and cooling properties helping flush kidneys and lymph system. And the fiber sweeps waste out through daily bowel movements.

Feel free to substitute seasonal ingredients or customize flavors based on your preferences!

Cleansing Salad Base

- Mixed greens – spinach, arugula, romaine, watercress, lettuces

- Chopped crucifers – broccoli, cabbage, brussels sprouts, kale

- Grated roots – carrots, beets, sweet potato

- Chopped alliums – onion, garlic, scallions

- Fresh herbs – cilantro, parsley, basil, mint

Antioxidant Berry Salad

Salad:

- 5 cups mixed baby greens

- 1/2 cup blackberries

- 1/2 cup raspberries

- 1/2 cup blueberries

- 1/4 cup pomegranate arils

Dressing:

- 3 Tbsp olive oil

- 1 Tbsp lemon juice

- 1 tsp maple syrup

- 1/4 tsp sea salt

- Crack of black pepper

Toss greens and berries with dressing just before serving. Top with crushed walnuts.

Benefits – liver support, skin cleansing, hydrating

Per serving: 250 cal | 4g P | 17g C | 19g F | 6g fiber

Cruciferous Detox Salad

Salad:

- 5 cups chopped kale

- 1/2 head broccoli, chopped

- 1/2 head cabbage, shredded

- 4 brussels sprouts, shredded

- 1 large carrot, grated

- 1/4 cup pumpkin seeds

Dressing:

- 3 Tbsp tahini

- 1 Tbsp olive oil

- 1 lemon, juiced

- 1" ginger, minced

- 1 garlic clove, minced

Toss salad with dressing right before eating.

Benefits – liver cleansing, gut support

Per serving: 380 cal | 12g P | 30g C | 27g F | 12g fiber

Hydrating Celery Cucumber Salad

Salad:

- 4 celery stalks, sliced

- 1 cucumber, sliced

- 1 cup strawberries, quartered

- 1 avocado, cubed

- 1/4 cup cilantro, chopped

Dressing:

- Juice of 2 limes

- 1 Tbsp olive oil

- 1 Tbsp maple syrup

- 1 tsp chili powder

- 1/4 tsp sea salt

Toss salad ingredients with dressing just before eating.

Benefits – kidney cleansing, cooling, hydrating

Per serving: 320 cal | 4g P | 30g C | 24g F | 10g fiber

Chapter 20: Soups and Broths

Warm, nourishing soups and broths comfort your body while flooding cells with minerals and fluids to promote detoxification. The heat stimulates digestion and absorption of nutrients to bolster cleansing pathways.

Broths also leach minerals from veggie cuts and bones into a mineral-rich, electrolyte cocktail your kidneys crave. Soup on!

Healing Miso Vegetable Soup

- 1 Tbsp coconut oil
- 3 garlic cloves, minced
- 1 onion, diced
- 3 carrots, diced
- 4 celery stalks, sliced
- 1 zucchini, chopped
- 8 cups water
- 1 cup diced cabbage
- 3" ginger, minced
- 4 Tbsp chickpea miso paste
- Juice from 1 lemon
- 4 cups chopped spinach
- Toasted sesame oil to finish

Sauté garlic, onion, carrots and celery 5 minutes. Add water, cabbage, ginger and miso dissolving as it simmers 10 minutes.

Remove from heat and stir in lemon juice, spinach till wilted. Drizzle sesame oil before serving.

Benefits – anti-inflammatory, liver and kidney support

Per serving: 150 cal | 6g P | 28g C | 3g F | 7g fiber

Mineralizing Bone Broth

- 3 lbs beef marrow bones
- 2 onions, roughly chopped
- 3 carrots, roughly chopped
- 3 celery stalks, roughly chopped
- 1 Tbsp ACV
- 2 bay leaves
- 5 peppercorns
- 1 Tbsp sea salt
- Water to cover bones
- Sprinkle fresh parsley before serving

Add bones, onion, carrots and celery to pot. Cover with water and add remaining ingredients except parsley. Bring to boil then reduce to simmer for 24-48 hours, skimming fat and adding water as reduces. Strain out solids once cooled and sprinkle parsley before drinking.

Benefits – hydrating, mineralizing, joint support

Per serving: 150 cal | 15g P | 6g C | 6g F | 2g fiber

Cleansing Turmeric Lentil Soup

- 1 Tbsp olive oil

- 1 onion, diced

- 3 garlic cloves, minced

- 1" ginger, minced

- 1 Tbsp turmeric

- 1 cup green or brown lentils, rinsed

- 6 cups vegetable broth

- 2 large carrots, chopped

- 3 celery stalks, chopped

- 1 (15oz) can diced tomatoes

- Juice of 1 lemon

- Chopped cilantro for garnish

Heat oil in pot over medium heat. Sauté onion, garlic and ginger 3 minutes until fragrant. Add turmeric and stir 30 seconds until fragrant. Add lentils, broth, carrots, celery and tomatoes. Bring to boil then cover and simmer 25 minutes until lentils are tender. Remove from heat and stir in lemon juice. Serve garnished with cilantro.

Benefits – anti-inflammatory, liver cleansing

Per serving: 230 cal | 16g P | 36g C | 3g F | 16g fiber

Chapter 21: Main Dishes

Center your lunch and dinner plates around clean proteins like wild caught fish or grass-fed meats alongside a medley of roasted, steamed or sautéed veggies. These complete meals provide balanced nutrition to nourish organs and pathways actively filtering toxins.

Explore herbs, spices and marinades to amplify nutritional content and flavor. Let's get cooking!

Citrus Baked Salmon

- 1.5 lbs wild salmon filet

- Zest of 1 orange

- Juice of 1 lemon

- 2 Tbsp olive oil

- 2 garlic cloves, minced

- 1 tsp dried oregano

- 1/2 tsp sea salt

- Lemon slices

Preheat oven 400°F. Place salmon skin-side down in baking dish. Mix orange zest, lemon juice, olive oil, garlic and oregano then pour over salmon. Sprinkle on sea salt.

Bake 15 minutes until just opaque and flakes easily. Garnish with lemon slices.

Benefits – anti-inflammatory, omega-3s, mineralizing

Per serving: 380 cal | 40g P | 2g C | 24g F | 0g fiber

Turmeric Roasted Cauliflower

- 1 large head cauliflower, cut into florets

- 1/4 cup olive oil

- 1 Tbsp turmeric

- 1 lemon, juiced

- 4 garlic cloves, minced

- 1 tsp sea salt

- 1/2 tsp black pepper

- 1/4 cup parsley, chopped

Preheat oven to 425°F. Toss cauliflower florets with olive oil, turmeric, lemon juice, garlic, salt and pepper until thoroughly coated. Spread on baking sheet in single layer.

Roast 30 minutes, flipping halfway through. Toss with parsley before serving. Enjoy!

Benefits – liver cleansing, anti-inflammatory

Per serving: 210 cal | 6g P | 13g C | 16g F | 6g fiber

Apple Cinnamon Quinoa Porridge

- 1 cup quinoa, rinsed

- 2 cups water or nut milk

- 1 apple, chopped

- 1 Tbsp almond butter

- 1 Tbsp maple syrup

- 1 tsp cinnamon

- 1/4 cup raisins

- Chopped walnuts to top

Add quinoa and water/milk to saucepan. Bring to boil, then cover and reduce to simmer 15 minutes until fluffy and water absorbed.

Remove from heat and stir in remaining ingredients. Enjoy porridge warm topped with walnuts.

Benefits – gluten free, blood sugar balance

Per serving: 490 cal | 12g P | 86g C | 12g F | 8g fiber

Chapter 22: Snacks

When detoxing, it's essential to keep blood sugar balanced through smaller, frequent feedings to prevent energy crashes, cravings or overeating.

Packing portable mini meals ensures you've got nourishing options on hand for between-meal bites. Choose snacks combining fiber, protein and healthy fats over quick-burning carbs.

Here are satiating staples for desk drawers, cars, bags and fridges!

Chia Fruit To-Go

- 1/2 cup diced berries
- 1/2 cup diced melon
- 2 Tbsp chia seeds
- 1/4 cup coconut milk

Mix together diced fruit, chia seeds and coconut milk in portable container with lid. Refrigerate overnight allowing to thicken into chia pudding. Enjoy!

Benefits – hydrating, fiber-rich, blood sugar

Per serving: 180 cal | 5g P | 25g C | 8g F | 12g fiber

Zesty Salsa Guacamole

- 2 medium avocados, cubed
- Juice from 1 lime
- 1 tomato, diced
- 1/4 cup cilantro, chopped
- 1/4 cup red onion, minced

- 1 garlic cloves, minced

- 1 jalapeño, ribs removed and minced

- 1/4 tsp sea salt

Gently combine all ingredients in bowl, mashing slightly to desired chunky texture. Scoop with sliced veggies or, nut crackers or bread.

Benefits – healthy fats, vitamin C, fiber

Per serving: 250 cal | 3g P | 13g C | 23g F | 8g fiber

Mediterranean Veggie Plate

- Celery sticks

- Carrot sticks

- Cucumber slices

- Red bell pepper slices

- Broccoli and cauliflower florets

- Olives

- 1/4 cup hummus

Arrange raw vegetable sticks and florets on plate. Place olives and hummus in center for dipping. Enjoy!

Benefits – hydrating vegetables, plant protein

Per serving: 180 cal | 7g P | 25g C | 6g F | 9g fiber

Apple Nachos

- 2 green apples, sliced into wedges

- 1/4 cup almond butter

- 1 Tbsp honey or maple syrup

- 1 Tbsp unsweetened coconut

- 1 tsp cinnamon

- 1/4 cup blueberries

Arrange apple wedges on plate like nachos. Drizzle with almond butter and honey/syrup. Sprinkle on coconut flakes and cinnamon. Top with a handful of blueberries. Dig in!

Benefits – balanced sweet snack, antioxidants

Per serving: 370 cal | 7g P | 49g C | 18g F | 7g fiber

Chapter 23: Desserts

Curb any sweet tooth cravings post cleanse with healthier, naturally-sweetened treats using detox-friendly ingredients. Date paste, maple syrup and almond flour step in for refined sugar, wheat flour and dairy to nurture your body rather than spike blood sugar or cause inflammation.

Incorporate soothing spices like cinnamon, vanilla, ginger and cardamom to stabilize energy levels after indulging your craving for something sweet!

Berry Chia Pudding

- 1 cup nut milk

- 2 Tbsp chia seeds

- 1/2 cup mixed berries

- 1 Tbsp maple syrup

- 1/2 tsp vanilla extract

- Pinch cinnamon

Whisk together nut milk, chia seeds, berries, maple syrup, vanilla and cinnamon in a bowl or mason jars. Refrigerate overnight to set. Top with additional berries before enjoying.

Benefits – fiber, omega-3's, antioxidants

Per serving: 180 cal | 5g P | 25g C | 6g F | 4g fiber

Carrot Cake Bites

- 1 cup almond flour

- 1/4 tsp sea salt

- 1/2 tsp baking soda

- 2 tsp cinnamon

- 3 eggs

- 1/4 cup coconut oil, melted

- 1/4 cup maple syrup

- 1 tsp vanilla extract

- 1 cup carrots, finely grated

- 1/2 cup walnuts, chopped

Preheat oven to 350°F. Mix together almond flour, salt, baking soda and cinnamon. Whisk in eggs, oil, maple syrup and vanilla until smooth batter forms. Fold in carrots and walnuts.

Scoop tablespoon sized bites onto parchment lined baking sheet. Bake 10 minutes until set. Enjoy!

Benefits – gluten free, blood sugar balance

Per serving: 180 cal | 6g P | 7g C | 15g F | 3g fiber

Dairy-Free Lemon Cheesecake

Crust:

- 1 1/2 cups almond flour

- 1/4 cup coconut oil

- 3 Tbsp maple syrup

- 1/2 lemon, zested

Filling:

- 2 (13.5oz) cans full-fat coconut milk, refrigerated overnight

- 1/3 cup lemon juice

- 1⁄3 cup maple syrup

- 2 Tbsp tapioca flour

- 2 tsp vanilla extract

- 1 lemon, zested

Process all crust ingredients in food processor until thick dough forms. Press into bottom of 8" springform pan. Refrigerate.

Scoop thick coconut cream layer off chilled cans (not watery liquid) into mixer. Add remaining filling ingredients beating until smooth, about 2 minutes. Pour filling onto crust. Refrigerate at least 6 hours to set. Garnish with fresh berries before slicing.

Benefits – probiotics, fiber, vitamin C

Per serving: 300 cal | 4g P | 15g C | 27g F | 3g fiber

Chapter 24: Juices and Tonics

Sipping on fresh pressed produce provides an influx of vitamins, minerals and phytonutrients in their most bioavailable form without taxing digestion. Combine cleansing fruits and vegetables into nutrient cocktails.

Botanical tonics also stimulate specific detox organs or pathways with their concentrated compounds. Take a shot daily!

Beet Ginger Detox Juice

- 5 carrots, greens removed
- 2 apples
- 1 lime, peeled
- 1 beet, greens removed
- 1" ginger root

Run all ingredients through a juicer. Stir to combine and serve over ice.

Benefits – liver stimulating, anti-inflammatory

Per serving: 230 cal | 4g P | 57g C | 1g F | 10g fiber

Hydrating Cucumber Mint Water

- 2 cucumbers, sliced
- 1 cup pineapple, cubed
- 1 lemon, sliced
- 5 fresh mint leaves
- Ice cubes

- Lime wedges for serving

Muddle cucumber, lemon and mint leaves in a pitcher, bruising to release oils and juice. Add pineapple chunks and stir in 4 cups filtered water. Allow to infuse in fridge at least 2 hours. Serve in glasses over ice with lime wedges.

Benefits – cooling, hydrating, alkalizing

Per serving: 40 cal | 1g P | 10g C | 0g F | 2g fiber

Metabolism Tonic Shot

- 2" ginger root, peeled

- Juice of 1 lemon

- Juice of 1 grapefruit

- 2 Tbsp ACV

- 1/8 tsp cayenne pepper

- 8 oz filtered water

Juice the ginger, lemon and grapefruit. Pour into glass jar with ACV and cayenne. Fill remainder of jar with water. Stir well and drink immediately. Rinse with extra water. Repeat daily.

Benefits – anti-inflammatory, lymphatic stimulant

Per serving: 35 cal | 1g P | 10g C | 0g F | 1g fiber Here is a draft Chapter 24 on Juices and Tonics for the recipe section of the book in markdown format:

Conclusion and Next Steps

Congratulations on completing The New Cleanse 21-day detox program! You have now guided your body through a gentle, yet deep cellular cleanse by supporting normal organ function and elimination routes. That is an incredible feat you should feel proud of.

As toxins accumulated over years steadily exit your system, improved energy, vitality, mental clarity and overall wellbeing should start setting in. With patience and continued self-care through proper eating, supportive lifestyle adjustments and addressing potential cleansing reactions, the gains you make during this program can continue unfolding in the weeks and months ahead.

However, the work does not stop with the final day of active cleansing! The ultimate goal is to carry forward the healthy lifestyle habits and patterns established so they become second nature. With commitment to the New Cleanse principles as your "new normal," your body will reach an even greater level of balance, efficiency and vibrancy.

So where do you go from here? **This concluding chapter is designed to send you forward equipped with all the tools, resources and motivation needed to continue your cleansing success long term.** We will recap:

- Key lessons and takeaways

- Lifestyle integration tips

- Further learning resources

- Finally, additional cleansing support options if desired

Use this conclusion as a reference to cement all that you have learned and achieved as you steadily deepen positive changes made during your program.

Key Lessons and Takeaways

- **Your body has an incredible, inborn detoxification intelligence** centered around the liver, kidneys, digestive organs and lymphatic system. Supporting normal organ function and elimination routes allows this elegant system to filter cellular waste and toxins effectively all on its own through nature's brilliant design!

- **Food as medicine** truly lies at the foundation of a cleansing lifestyle. Nourishing your detox organs and pathways with strategic, whole foods gives your body exactly what it needs to reset toxicity accumulated over time and restore itself back into balance effortlessly and completely naturally.

- **Reducing everyday toxin exposures** further allows your body's natural detox process to focus inward rather than constantly defending against chemical inputs from outside. Limiting avoidable toxins in your living environment dramatically lightens the load.

- **Actively supporting elimination functions** through quick daily rituals essentially gives your exit hatches for accumulated waste a beneficial nudge - further enhancing your body's self-regulating detox capabilities exponentially.

- **Patience and self-compassion is vital** while cleansing as well as maintaining changes long-term. Progress happens in layers with ups and downs along the way. Trust your body's intuitive wisdom to balance and renew itself in due time through consistent care.

If you continue respecting your body's ideal state through the New Cleanse approach, vibrancy and balance can become your normal! Health is your body's default when properly supported.

Lifestyle Integration Tips

In order to make this clean, toxin-free lifestyle second nature going forward, adopt the 80/20 principle outlined in Chapter 16:

- **80% of the time** strictly follow the New Cleanse diet principles, activity recommendations, toxin avoidance habits and general healthy protocols

- **20% of the time** loosen up for special occasions, weekends or holidays

Also continue implementing key supporting practices daily:

- Upon rising - Hot lemon water, dry brush skin, oil pulling

- Morning - Elimination rituals, meditation, movement

- Throughout day - Skin brushing, hydration, clean eating

- Evening - Lymph drainage practices, relaxation, early bedtime

Additionally, surround yourself with positive community and accountability systems to reinforce new habits. Share your wins, challenges and lessons learned with friends, family and practitioners committed to healthy clean-living principles too.

Following these practical steps makes integration after completing a program infinitely easier while cementing positive changes made!

Further Learning Resources

While this guide aims to provide a comprehensive overview on effectively supporting your body's innate detoxification processes for full cleansing and restoration, there is always more to learn!

Here are some suggested resources if you wish to deepen your knowledge on core topics covered:

Cleansing and Detoxification

- *The Detox Prescription* by Woodson Merrell, MD

- *The Elimination Diet* by Tom Malterre

- *Clean Gut* by Alejandro Junger, MD

- *Medical Medium Liver Rescue* by Anthony William

- *The Cleansing Program* by Dr. Richard Anderson

Herbs and Supplements

- *Herbal Medicine Natural Remedies* by Dr. Christopher Hobbs

- *Adaptogens: Herbs for Strength, Stamina and Stress Relief* by David Winston

- *The Neti Pot for Better Health* by Warren Jefferson

Gut Health Digestion

- *Eat for Life* by Dr. Joseph Mercola

- *The Bountiful Benefits of Bone Broth* by Allison Siebecker

- *Gut and Psychology Syndrome* by Natasha Campbell-McBride

Explore which body systems need further nutritional support or which cleansing modalities most call to you. Tailor your learning journey as your needs evolve!

Additional Cleansing Support Options

If after completing The New Cleanse program, you find certain symptoms or toxicity still lingering needing additional targeted support, consider one of the following:

Professional Cleansing Programs – Several resorts, detox centers and practitioner offices offer supervised cleanse programs to reset specific organ systems:

- Liver and full body cleansing

- Kidney and lymphatic drainage

- Digestive repair and gut cleansing

- Anti-parasitic, antibacterial eradication

Juice Fasting – For a more intensive cellular reset, commit to a vegetable juicing fast for 3-7 days while eliminating solid foods under supervision of your physician.

Intermittent Fasting – Also effective for cellular rejuvenation, fasting windows from 12-72 hours allows metabolic waste and toxins to filter out while triggering autophagy and stem cell production once stores are depleted.

Advanced Testing - Specialized lab testing analyzes specific toxin levels, metal exposures, digestive pathogens or system dysfunctions needing custom repair:

- Heavy metal, mold or chemical panels

- Organic acid test

- Comprehensive stool analysis

- Food sensitivity testing

Reaching out for professional support designing a targeted treatment plan for lingering symptoms makes cleansing more efficient by personalizing protocols to your unique biochemistry, sensitivities and needs.

I sincerely hope The New Cleanse has guided you to profoundly improve wellness through supporting your body's elegant detoxification capabilities. Remember that vibrancy is your natural state when properly nourished! I wish you abundant energy and resilience on your continued health journey ahead.

Warmly,

Dr. Omolola Habib (NMD)

About the Author

I'm Dr. Omolola Habib, a passionate naturopathic doctor, holistic nutritionist, and wellness advocate. My mission is to empower people to achieve optimal health through transformative yet gentle detox protocols that harness the body's innate healing wisdom.

For over a decade, I've helped numerous individuals overhaul their wellbeing by addressing root causes of imbalance, rather than just treating symptoms. My specialty is creating personalized cleansing programs focused on dietary strategies, toxin avoidance, lifestyle changes, and natural remedies tailored to each person.

I firmly believe that vibrant health is our natural state when the mind, body and spirit are nourished synergistically. This whole-person approach is central to my practice philosophy and permeates the guidance I share.

As author of "The New Cleanse: A Fresh Restorative Program for Full Body Detoxification," I translate years of clinical experience into an accessible resource. My goal is to expand vital knowledge so more people can embrace the benefits of detoxification to revitalize energy and resilience from within.

I feel immensely grateful for opportunities supporting individuals on their journey toward holistic healing and prevention. With compassion plus practical wisdom, I continue impacting lives through regenerative naturopathic solutions reconnecting clients to their inner thriving self once more.

www.ingramcontent.com/pod-product-compliance
Lightning Source LLC
Chambersburg PA
CBHW070851260726
48661CB00004B/1347